AN INTRODUCTION TO ORIENTAL DIAGNOSIS

Your Face Never Lies

Michio Kushi

Edited by
William Tara and David Lasocki
Illustrated by David Elliott

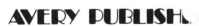

AVERY PUBLISH.
Wayne, New Jersey

The medical and health procedures in this book are based on the training, personal experiences and research of the author. Because each person and situation is unique, the editor and publisher urge the reader to check with a qualified health professional before using any procedure where there is any question as to its appropriateness.

The publisher does not advocate the use of any particular diet and exercise program, but believes the information presented in this book should be available to the public.

Because there is always some risk involved, the author and publisher are not responsible for any adverse effects or consequences resulting from the use of any of the suggestions, preparations, or procedures in this book. Please do not use the book if you are unwilling to assume the risk. Feel free to consult a physician or other qualified health professional. It is a sign of wisdom, not cowardice, to seek a second or third opinion.

Originally published in the United Kingdom by Red Moon Press, 1976, a division of Sunwheel Foods Ltd., London, England.

Cover photograph by Kathryn Abbe
Cover designed by Rudy Shur and Martin Hochberg

Printed in the United States of America

10 9 8 7 6 5 4 3 2 1

Contents

Preface

Accurate diagnosis is a key factor in the treatment of any illness. With clear knowledge of the major symptoms, a cure is easily sought. Modern medical diagnosis often employs techniques such as exploratory surgery or the administration of dyes followed by X-rays, all of which can actually harm the patient; and it seems that the more specialized these techniques become, the greater their potential risk. Moreover, these sophisticated forms of diagnosis look only at the body, its function, and its physiology, while attempting to pinpoint the cause of the problem. The person's overall health, mental state, and lifestyle are completely, and quite mistakenly, overlooked. Perhaps this inadequacy of modern diagnosis explains the relative failure of medicine—and the success of wholistic therapies such as macrobiotics—in reversing degenerative illnesses including cancer.

Oriental diagnosis views the total person, physically and mentally, as well as the troubled organs or body parts. The practitioner interprets the person's lifestyle and social and environmental surroundings to arrive at the cause and cure of the problem. Traditionally this wholistic diagnosis was used not only to study individuals, but to analyze society as well. It was passed on by word of mouth only, having its origin in the Oriental law of change as indicated in *The Book of Changes* (I-Ching) and other Oriental classics.

Without books or schools from which to gain knowledge, my own understanding of Oriental diagnosis developed slowly, only after years of practice. The late George Oshawa, a philosopher and expert in Oriental medicine, directed me to the study of biology, biochemistry, astronomy, history, and other scientific and cultural disciplines so that I could obtain an understanding of human health and illness—and ultimatly a humane and effective form of diagnosis.

Thanks to the efforts of William Tara, who edited the lectures that gave birth to this book, you can begin learning the basics of Oriental diagnosis in a matter of days, for diagnostic skills are useful not only for medical practitioners but for anyone who wishes to refine his awareness of those around him.

Oriental diagnosis requires neither expensive equipment nor elaborate technology. Your eyes, ears, touch, nose, and intuition are the only tools employed. Of course, the sharper your instruments—the healthier you are—the more accurate your perceptions will be. Therefore, I recommend that you refine your own health and sensitivity as I have, by adopting a wholesome macrobiotic diet consisting mainly of whole grains, beans and vegetables.

I sincerely hope that this introductory book will stimulate further study. My book, *How to See Your Health: Book of Oriental Diagnosis* (Japan Publications) and regular articles appearing in the EastWest Journal are recommended for further reading. Through regaining a sensitivity to your own body, and better understanding the health of your loved ones, friends and associates, you can learn to recognize the signs of physical illness, and prevent—even reverse—its development, while restoring vibrant health.

Michio Kushi

Ackowledgements

The material contained in this book was taken from lectures given by Michio Kushi between 1970 and 1973 at the East West Foundation in Boston, Massachusetts. The material as finally developed constituted a seminar entitled "Diagnosis and Physiognomy," held in April and May 1973 and published in the *Michio Kushi Seminar Report*, Volume III, Nos. 1-4, edited by Jim Ledbetter. Some additional material appeared in *The Order of the Universe*, Volume IV, Nos. 7 and 10, edited by Thomas Lloyd.

We are highly indebted to Mr. Kushi for his encouragement and support in producing this book. We would also like to thank Jim Ledbetter and Thomas Lloyd for their work in the original transcription of the material. A special word of appreciation must go to Sherman Goldman for his generosity in reading the manuscript of the book and making many helpful suggestions.

Introduction

Oriental Diagnosis

The medicine of China, Japan and other countries of the Far East is among the oldest in the world. This medicine can teach us a great deal that can be practically applied today. The basic philosophy of Oriental medicine is the complementary opposite of the kind of medicine currently practised in the West. Western medicine, with its emphasis on the treatment of symptoms by drugs and surgery, is increasingly powerless to cope with the rising tide of degenerative illness that now threatens to engulf the industrialised world. Clearly we need to supplement our mainly symptomatic medicine with a medicine that is preventive in direction and humane and economical in application. Oriental medicine can contribute greatly to filling this need.

The standard Oriental writings on the causes of disease stressed the relationship between an individual's health and his or her diet, activity, spiritual attitude and total environment. No single aspect of human life was considered separate from another. The biological, psychological and spiritual were seen as related aspects of the totality. The practitioner was an adviser and teacher who could point out the source of a health problem and give practical suggestions for changes in life style that could ameliorate the problem at its source.

In Western medicine, diagnosis identifies a disease by observation of its symptoms. The experienced Oriental diagnostician, however, can foresee the development of sickness before the sick person has specific symptoms such as pain. The principal tool of Oriental diagnosis is physiognomy — the art of judging a person "from the features of the face or the form and lineaments of the body generally" (Oxford English Dictionary). The basic premise of Oriental physiognomy is that each individual represents a walking history of his or her development. The strengths and weaknesses of our parents, the environment we were brought up in, and the food we have eaten are all expressed in our present condition. Our posture, the colour of our skin, the tone of our voice and other traits are externalisations of the condition of our blood, organs, nervous system, and skeletal structure, which in turn are the result of our heredity, diet, environment, and activity.

The secret of diagnostic skill is to recognise the signs of a particular set of changes before they become serious — to see the signs that stones are developing in the kidneys, that the heart is becoming expanded, or that a cancer is developing — even before these symptoms bring pain and discomfort. This type of diagnosis depends completely on the practitioner developing his or her own sensitivity and understanding fully the principles that underlie the techniques.

Yin and Yang

The principle behind Oriental medicine is the theory of yin and yang. The starting premise of yin/yang philosophy is that everything in the universe exists in a continual state of change. This change is expressed in terms of yin becoming yang or yang becoming yin. Yin and yang are relative, not absolute. Everything exists in complementary opposition. Without cold there would be no hot; without up there would be no down. Without opposition there would be no movement, no change. As the *Tao Te Ching* puts it, "From the One came Two, and from the Two all things were born".

If the tendency of any movement is contracting, or moving towards a centre, then the dominant force is yang. Contraction produces density, activity, heat, weight, speed, etc. If the tendency is expansion, or moving away from a centre, then the dominant force is yin. Dispersion produces less density, less activity, lightness, slower speed, etc. At the extremes, yin and yang change into one another. Contraction at the limiting point produces a tendency to expand, and vice versa.

This pulse of life governs all things, from the way the tides ebb and flow and plants grow by a sequence of integration and differentiation, to the yearly pattern of the planets around the sun. Within our body we are aware of the expansion and contraction of the heart, the filling and emptying of the lungs, and the tension and relaxation of the muscles.

From the ancient philosophy of yin and yang, George Ohsawa extracted seven principles and twelve theorems that summarise the operation of these forces. If the reader wishes to have a real understanding of the material of this book, we strongly advise him or her to study these principles and theorems. Without such understanding, the particular techniques are of almost no value.

The Seven Principles of the Order of the Universe

1. All things are the differentiation of One Infinity.
2. Everything changes.
3. All antagonisms are complementary.
4. There is nothing identical.
5. Whatever has a front has a back.
6. The bigger the front the bigger the back.
7. Whatever has a beginning has an end.

The Twelve Theorems of the Unifying Principle

1. One Infinity differentiates into yin and yang, which are the poles created when the infinite centrifugality arrives at the geometric point of bifurcation.
2. Yin and yang result continuously from this infinite centrifugality.
3. Yin is centrifugal. Yang is centripetal. Yin and yang together produce energy and all phenomena.
4. Yin attracts yang. Yang attracts yin.
5. Yin repels yin. Yang repels yang.
6. The force of repulsion is proportional to the difference between the like components, and the force of attraction is proportional to the difference between the unlike components.
7. All phenomena are ephemeral, constantly changing their constitution of yin and yang components.
8. Everything involves polarity. Nothing is solely yin or solely yang.
9. There is nothing neutral. In every occurrence either yin or yang is in excess.
10. Large yin attracts small yin. Large yang attracts small yang.
11. At their extremes, yin produces yang, and yang produces yin.
12. All physical forms and objects are yang at the centre and yin at the surface.

	YIN	YANG
motion	expansion	contraction
category	space	time
position	outward	inward
direction	ascent	descent
colour	purple, blue, green	yellow, orange, red
temperature	cold	hot
weight	light	heavy
catalyst	water	fire
light	bright	dark
vibration	short wave	long wave
atomic particle	electron	proton
elements	K, O, P, Ca, N, etc.	H, As, Cl, Na, C, etc.
biology	vegetable	animal
sex	female	male
nervous system	orthosympathetic	parasympathetic
attitude	gentle, negative	active, positive
activity	psychological	physical
origin	hot climate	cold climate

Yin and Yang and the Classification of the Organs

The classification of organs into yin and yang used in this book is opposite to that found in some books on acupuncture. The system used here is based on the *structure* of the organ. In this book, organs that are more solid and dense, such as the heart, liver, spleen, etc., are classified as yang; organs that are hollow, such as the stomach, bladder, intestines, etc., are classified as yin. The classification used in some acupuncture books refers to the quality of "Ch'i" energy that forms and nourishes the organs.

In Oriental medicine each major organ is considered to be in an antagonistic/complementary relationship with another major organ, as follows:

Lungs . . . . Large Intestines
Heart. . . . . .Small Intestines
Kidneys. . . . .(Urinary) Bladder
Spleen . . . . .Stomach
Liver . . . . .Gall Bladder

If any problem arises in one organ of the pair, there will also be a problem with the complementary organ.

Diet and Diagnosis

According to Oriental medicine, proper diet is the principal source of our vitality and health; a poor diet is the principal cause of sickness. If our diet does not enable us to respond to changes in the climate and our activity as we develop, then sickness arises. A proper diet should reflect the evolution of humanity, the environment the individual is living in and the type of activity he or she is engaged in.

The tools for discovering our proper diet, and how we can vary that to fit our personal needs, are yin and yang. To understand the importance of yin and yang in food selection we can look at the yearly cycle of vegetal energy. Plants grow in complementary opposition to their climate. That is, if the climate is yang, yin plants are produced, and vice versa. In the winter it is cold (yin). During this time of year the energy in the vegetal world descends to the roots of plants (yang). In the summer it is hot (yang); the energy of the plant is drawn up and out (yin). Winter vegetables, such as parsnips and pumpkin, are drier, grow slowly and are heavy. Summer plants, such as lettuce and cucumber, grow quickly, have more water and are generally light. If we eat the foods that grow in the season and location in which we are living, we also can make balance with our natural environment. Thus, Bedouin, for example, eat the juicy fruit (yin) of cacti which grow in the dry (yang) desert. Eskimos live almost entirely off meat (yang) to provide them with warmth in their cold (yin) climate.

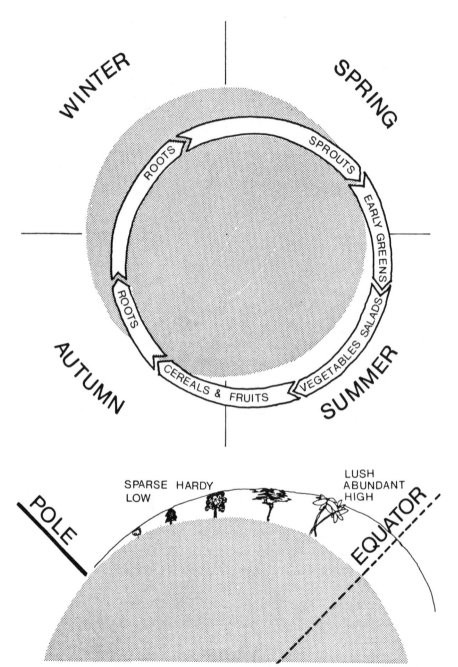

The cycle of vegetal energy and its relationship to the seasons and climate.

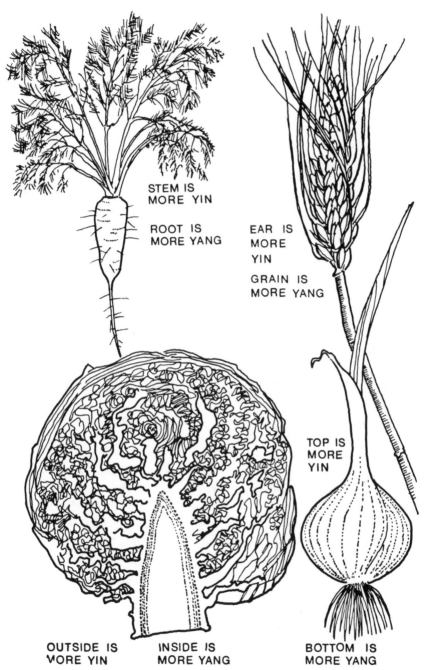

STEM IS
MORE YIN

ROOT IS
MORE YANG

EAR IS
MORE
YIN

GRAIN IS
MORE YANG

TOP IS
MORE
YIN

OUTSIDE IS
MORE YIN

INSIDE IS
MORE YANG

BOTTOM IS
MORE YANG

Several common food plants and the yin and yang factors in their structure.

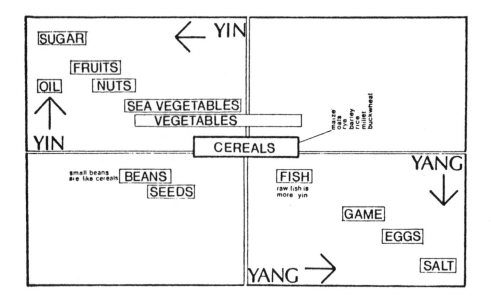

Using the principles of yin and yang in food selection and preparation is an important part of 'macrobiotics', a word adopted by George Ohsawa to describe Oriental dietary and medical principles to the West. It is a combination of 'macro', meaning great or large, and 'biotic', meaning related to life or living things. Macrobiotics is a way of making our life larger, more in touch with the environment, closer to the infinite. Through regaining our sensitivity to the environment we can begin to experience our relationship with nature and our own ability to freely determine our health and destiny. An important tool in taking active responsibility for our health is Oriental diagnosis, which indicates the deficiencies or excesses in our diet. If we can recognise these signs we can then change the food we eat in an appropriate manner, reverse the course of developing sickness, and begin to restore our health.

David Lasocki
William Tara

Order and Method of Diagnosis

When diagnosing people, try to see their total condition, their wholeness. See their past, present and future — their background, their physical and mental condition, and their possibilities for growth. What is their destiny? Consider their personality, their judgement, and their spiritual level. The Order of Diagnosis comprises three steps. First, you understand the individual's total environment. Second, you see his present physical and mental condition and relate it to the totality. Third, you see the details — symptoms. Modern Western medicine tends to pass over the first two steps and concentrate on the third.

The Method of Diagnosis comprises five steps: (1) intuitively grasping the whole; (2) listening to the person's case history; (3) observing the person's handwriting or aesthetic expression; (4) seeing the symptoms; and (5) touching to confirm what you have seen. Work in this order; do not touch first. In this way you can develop your intuition. Then, even when people are not with you, you can know their condition by intuition. And when they come to see you, you will already have an image of them. You may not know the details, but you have a feeling about what their problem is.

You know this already from personal experience. When you meet strangers you have a feeling about their personality or their spirituality. When you check their symptoms by listening, seeing and touching, you are learning in more detail what you already know about them. By developing your sensitivity, you can diagnose even when the person only calls you on the telephone or writes you a letter. If you become really good, you do not have to meet people at all. Of course, people would not be satisfied with this, so we have to meet them. Still, sitting down with people, talking to them, touching, should be nothing but confirmation. This keen intuition is the essence of traditional Oriental medicine, but unfortunately most doctors — Oriental and Western — have lost this ability.

1

Let us consider the order and method of diagnosis in a little more detail. When first looking at people, ask yourself how old they are. Their chronological age is less important than their biological age. A person who is chronologically only eighteen may be much older than that physically and spiritually. Healthy people should look younger than average people their age. A twenty-year old should appear two to three years younger; a person of thirty years of age, three to four years younger; a person of forty, five years younger; and so on.

Next try to sense their level of mental evolution: do they seek spiritual things?; what is their scope of judgement? Then determine whether their development tends to be smooth or whether they have radical ups and downs. Are they orderly or disorderly? To see these tendencies, look at the side of the face. Many hollows, indentations and corresponding high places indicate a tendency to go to extremes.

You should also see in what kind of environment individuals were brought up: small city, big city, or the country. Is their way of life easy or hard? Are they rich or poor? For this you must study the bones. People brought up in a city are generally weaker than those brought up in the country. The fragility of their bones shows this long term weakness.

You can then begin to use this information to visualise individuals' past and future life. You should be able to see what is in store for them if they continue to live the way they are going.

As people become healthier, they tend to become more active socially. You can see if a person has the potential for leadership. The natural ability to lead is indicated by a strong constitution, large hands, and large ears that lie flat to the head.

After you have gained a general impression, it is time to look at the details. What kinds of foods has the person enjoyed, and what effects have these foods had on their health? Observe which organs are weak — the heart, spleen, large intestine — and check the effect of this weakness on the complementary organs (see p. xi). If the heart is weak, for instance, check the condition of the small intestine.

As an example, let us consider the spleen. To check for problems with the spleen look at the bony ridges above the eye and the periphery of the ear: they will be red. You can also see spleen problems on the sides of the bridge of the nose: there is often a slightly green colour.

2

Many people in the modern world have spleen problems caused by the removal of their tonsils. If the tonsils are removed, the spleen must work harder; there is more stress, and problems may develop. This is especially true when people consume sugar, chemicals or drugs. The removal of their tonsils decreases their resistance to the strain caused by the intake of those things. The spleen is a cleansing organ for the blood and the lymphatic system; the tonsils perform the same kind of function. Swollen tonsils indicate that toxic material is being gathered there. When we operate to remove the tonsils, we destroy this function and spread the toxins to other parts of the body.

The method of diagnosis taught in this book is an integral part of preventive medicine, which sees symptoms not as problems to be removed but as indications of underlying causes which can then be changed at their point of origin.

The Embryo

We must distinguish between people's *condition* and their *constitution*. Constitution is determined before birth — by the characteristics of the mother, father and ancestors, and by the food eaten by the mother during the individual's embryonic stage of development. The bone structure, the facial structure, the depth and width of the skull, the shape of the hands and feet, and to some extent the height and width of the body and the length of the legs — all these make up a person's constitution. The characteristics acquired later, such as the hue and texture of the skin, indicate a person's condition. It is relatively easy to change people's condition through good diet and other changes in life style, but it is almost impossible to change their constitution. What happens to the embryo during the mother's pregnancy is crucial for health and happiness.

Our body has three main systems: the digestive, the nervous, and the circulatory. The digestive system of the embryo is on the inside (yang) and the nervous system on the outside (yin). As both systems develop they gather to themselves opposite factors and therefore change polarity. Minerals go to the back, and proteins, fats, etc. go to the front. The yin outside of the body attracts yang and becomes hard, forming the spinal column and back. The yang inside attracts yin and becomes soft, forming the internal organs. This alteration is an excellent example of the fact that yin and yang are not static, but dynamic, always changing.

The lower portion of the digestive system, below the rib cage, handles the yang part of physical food (solids and liquids). The upper portion, above the rib cage, becomes the lungs, developing the capacity to handle yin physical food (air).

The nervous system is also divided into two. At the time in his evolution when Man was without consciousness, there was only one, undifferentiated nervous system, which had orthosympathetic characteristics. This then divided to form the central nervous system and the autonomic nervous system. Finally, the autonomic system further divided into orthosympathetic and parasympathetic systems. The orthosympathetic system makes yin organs expand and yang organs contract. The parasympathetic system makes yin organs contract and yang organs expand.

5

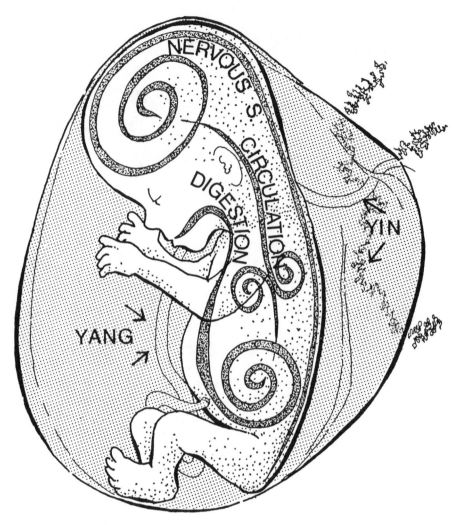

The relative position of the three major systems in the embryo

How can we divide the circulatory functions by yin and yang? Blood is red and active (yang). Lymph is clear and slowly gathers the used body fluid from the periphery and takes it back to the heart. These systems are again yin and yang, distributing and gathering.

In the body there are two major antagonisms — front and back. Solid, liquid and air are all taken in by the front systems (digestive and respiratory). Then vibrations — short ones, long ones, magnetic ones — are all taken in by the back system (nervous). Food, which is yang, is drawn downwards spirally and dispatched from the lower centre. Vibrations, which are yin, tend to go upwards, again in spiral motion, to the brain. Metaphysically, these two regions are called the 'hara' and 'third eye'. They should be kept warm and cool, yang and yin, respectively. If these front and back activities do not coordinate well, one cannot control food and nerve impulses.

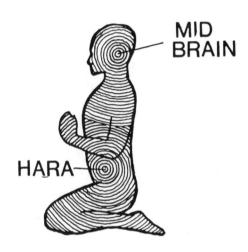

MID
BRAIN

HARA

The circulatory, digestive and nervous systems all gather at the region of the mouth. This region is the tightest place in the body, the most yang. Yang can gather and take in; from this region we eat and breathe. Yang is also active; from this region there is also movement — we talk. The mouth is the body's centre, the place where we exercise our consciousness and freedom. It is the pivot of the body's functioning. By controlling our eating, breathing and talking, we control our lives.

Whether the region of the mouth is yin or yang is the prime determining factor of each individual's personality or spirituality. This region is a clue to the whole body; we must learn to 'read' it. Look at your friends and see if their mouths are tightly closed or not, whether they are loose or swollen, etc.

The position of the embryo can be seen in the following drawing.

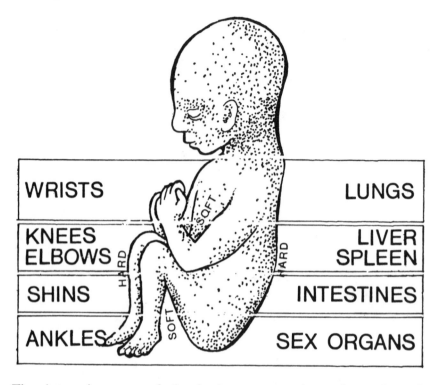

WRISTS		LUNGS
KNEES ELBOWS		LIVER SPLEEN
SHINS		INTESTINES
ANKLES		SEX ORGANS

The internal organs of the body correspond to the embryonic position of the arms and legs. The ankles and buttocks correspond to organs on that level — the sexual organs. The middle region of the legs corresponds to the digestive organs. The area around the knees and elbows corresponds to the liver, spleen and pancreas. The hands are folded across the chest. The wrist therefore corresponds to the organs at that level — the lungs. The hands can also be folded across the face. When we are startled or embarrassed or cry, our hand goes immediately to our face; we yangize and our hands take their embryonic position.

After birth, our arms hang at our sides and begin to have a correspondence with the areas to which they are now in proximity. The wrist area begins to represent the sexual functions. If our wrist is stiff, the energy in the sexual area is blocked, rigid. If the wrist is flexible, the sexual organs are functioning well.

You can observe the condition of people's bodies easily during the summer when they are wearing shorts or swimming costumes. Notice any marks, hair, spots, veins; observe where the body is expanded or tight; note the general colour. All year round, however, we can diagnose people's condition by giving them a massage. Are there any places on the legs, for instance, that are watery, tight, or swollen? Remember that the ankles represent the sex organs; the Achilles tendon should be tight. The calf represents the intestines, and higher up the leg shows the condition of the liver, spleen and pancreas.

If a person's spine is curved, then the organs at the level of the curvature are either swollen or tense. It is easy for the cartilage between the vertebrae to become expanded and out of line. Are the spaces between the vertebrae even or not? If there is a big space, the region behind this place is too yin — expanded by intake of sugar or excess liquid. If the space is too small, the region is too yang, tight — from excess meat or salt — but this condition is rare. If we push strongly in a place and there is pain, something is wrong in the corresponding organ.

The Face

No one has a perfectly proportioned body or head. Each of us is different, depending upon the foods we are nourished with while in our mother's womb. Facial proportions can tell us a great deal about a person's constitution, their condition at birth. We can divide the face into three sections, as shown in the diagram below.

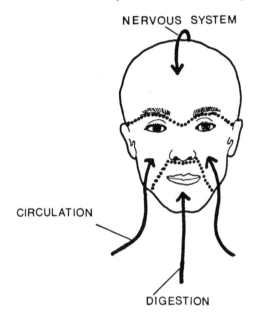

The three sections of the face and the development of the corresponding major systems of the body.

During the first seven days after conception the fertilised egg travels down the fallopian tube towards the depth of the womb where implantation occurs, and the organism increases rapidly in size for the next 21 days. These first 28 days account for the main development of the top section of the face. If chemicals or drugs are taken during this period there will be trouble for the person's whole life (less so if the drugs were taken before implantation). 'Birthmarks' are usually caused in this period. During the next 63 days the middle section of the face has its principal development. At 91 days all of the structures are generally formed. The bottom section of the face develops most during the remaining 189 days before gestation. Note that all the periods just mentioned — 7, 21, 63 and 189 days — increase in the proportion one to three.

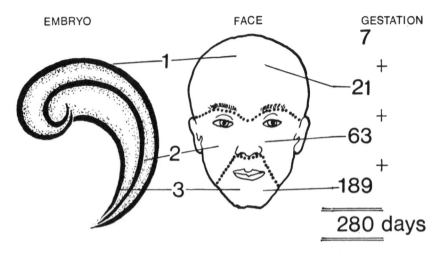

EMBRYO   FACE   GESTATION

$$7 + 21 + 63 + 189 \over 280 \text{ days}$$

The development of the systems in the embryo.

The three systems of the embryo develop continuously, but the principal development of each system takes place as follows. During the first three months the nervous system progresses rapidly. After this, during the second three months, the circulatory system and the organs used in filtering the blood and balancing go through a period of rapid development. The final three months see the greatest development within the respiratory and digestive systems. The most yang system (nervous) is developed at the periphery of the embryonic spiral (the most yin part). The digestive system, which is hollow (yin), develops at the centre of the spiral (the most yang position). In between these two systems, making balance, is the circulatory system.

Since pregnancy lasts nine months, we pass only three seasons in the womb. Our development takes place in four ways in relation to the seasons: spring, summer, autumn; summer, autumn, winter; autumn, winter, spring; and winter, spring, summer. In ancient times people ate more yang food in winter and more yin food in summer.

This led to contraction (yang) or expansion (yin) of the section of the face that was developing during the particular season. We can still look at people over the age of forty and see clearly which season they were born in. But since we now eat so many foods out of season — for instance, ice cream and bananas in winter — younger people have different proportions in the face.

Following traditional patterns of eating, there are four basic shapes of face that correspond to the four orders of seasons possible during pregnancy.

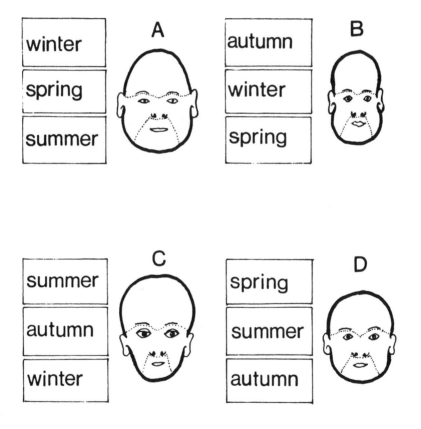

Type A is steady and practical. Type B is more romantic and emotional, sentimental, idealistic. Type C tends to be a thinker, intellectual. Type D is active, a do-er.

Constitution and Condition

All matter is created by a contracting force which reaches a limit of contraction and then expands. All material things therefore tend to be yang (dense) inside and yin outside. The stronger the contracting force, the greater the expanding force. The leaves in the diagram below are arranged to show the effect on their structure of decreased contraction due to increasingly hot climate. The leaf on the left is an evergreen from a northern area; the contracting force is great. The leaf on the right is from a tropical area; the expanding force is greater than the contracting force. The leaf in the middle, from a temperate climate, shows a balance of forces.

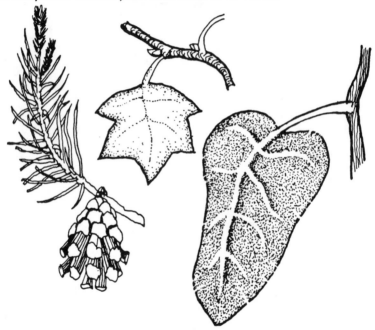

These trees are all affected by the climate and the nourishment they take from the soil. The internal and external forces strive for balance. It is the same with mankind. We receive influences from nature and society, and we generate our own internal force. All these affect our form. We cannot control the external forces, but we can control the internal force through our diet. As far as physical food is concerned, if we take in an excess of food or more yin food, our internal force is expansive. If we take in little food or more yang food, our internal force is more concentrated.

We can see the operation of the internal force in the features of the face. Some people's eyes are more indented (yang internal force), some are more protruding (yin). People who have flat noses cannot hold eyeglasses on; but since they are more yang they seldom need glasses. If you observe people on the streets you will notice that some have mouths that are swollen towards the outside; others have thin, shallow lips. The thin lipped people are usually strong, but often also tend to be inflexible.

The vertical direction is yin (expanding force away from the earth); the horizontal direction, yang. Long, narrow eyes are therefore more yang; wide eyes (with more vertical force), more yin. A long nose, especially one that protrudes, is yin; a flat nose is more yang. Horizontally expanded nostrils indicate a yang constitution. A large, well-defined jaw is another important sign of a yang constitution. People with such a horizontal form in their face are often very active.

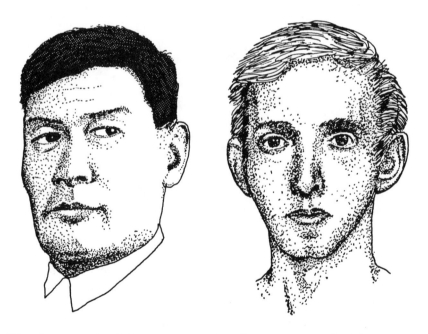

The face on the left is an example of a more yang facial structure. The face on the right is more yin, governed by vertical movement.

A person's constitution is established in the womb. Before birth the structure of the face is created. As far as the constitution is concerned, horizontal lines are a sign of yang. After birth, however, features such as wrinkles appear. Vertical expansion (yin) causes the skin to wrinkle in horizontal lines. Such wrinkles are most common on the forehead, where they are caused by excess liquid (yin).

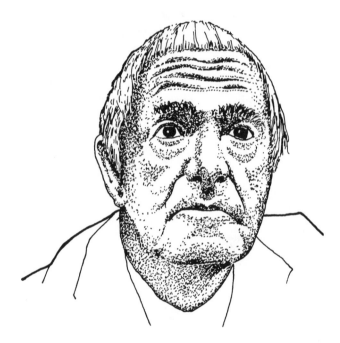

An example of horizontal lines on the face in the area of the forehead and under the eyes. These are caused by excess liquid, not the facial structure.

Vertical lines between the eyes indicate problems with the liver and gall bladder. Below the liver area, on either side of the nose, is the area corresponding to the spleen and pancreas — and, because these organs are complementary to the stomach, also corresponding to the stomach. The green colour often found in this region indicates problems with the stomach and spleen.

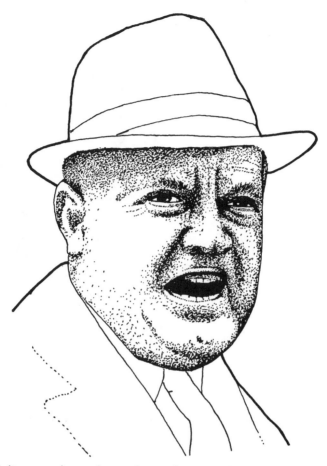

Vertical lines such as those above the nose, between the eyebrows, are caused by an excess of yang food in the diet. These lines are a sign of a bad liver.

Since the shape of the eyebrows is determined by the under-lying bone structure, it is an indication of the individual's constitution. If a mother eats more yang food, especially meat, while she is pregnant, the baby's eyebrows will be slanted down to-wards the middle of the face. Vegetarian peoples have eyebrows that are curved down towards the outside.

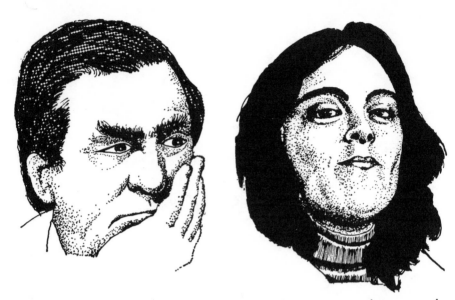

The face on the left has eyebrows which have a strong slant towards the centre. This is a sign of an intake of excess of animal foods. The face on the right has eyebrows which are more yin and curve towards the outside.

The length and thickness of the eyebrows are determined after birth. If you lose your eyebrows, they fall away from the outside. Long eyebrows are a sign of happiness and longevity. Thickness shows strong vitality; thin eyebrows are a sign of weak vitality.

The top of the face is a large cleft that reflects the structure of the brain. In the region of the nose and mouth there is a gathering of features (yang). The nose and mouth should be free from clefts, but we often see a cleft on the tip of the nose or on the lips. These show poor coordination between the two sides of the body. A cleft in the nose means that the two sides of the heart are not balancing, and there is a so-called heart murmur. People with such clefts have little stamina; they cannot run well. The condition usually dates from birth, but can be worsened through poor eating.

The extreme case of a cleft in the lips is the so-called hare lip. It is an indication of excess yin. It develops in the mother's womb when the food she is eating does not have enough yang power to complete the contracting force forming the face.

If a person's nose is swollen and looks soft and watery, it indicates that the heart is swollen from intake of too much liquid. If the swelling is fat and hard, it indicates sinus problems caused by an excess of butter and cheese in the diet. The area around the heart has fat deposits. People with this harder swelling are prone to heart attacks; the heart is swollen and therefore inflexible.

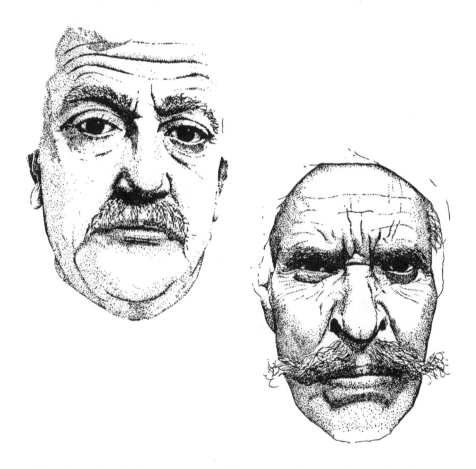

The lines in the face are caused by yin and yang forces. In the top figure we see the lines caused by yin (expansion) which has a tendency to go up and cause horizontal wrinkles. Sugars, fats and liquid can all be causes of these lines. The bottom figure shows the contracting yang force, which produces vertical wrinkles. This force can be caused by eating animal foods or excessive amounts of salt.

19

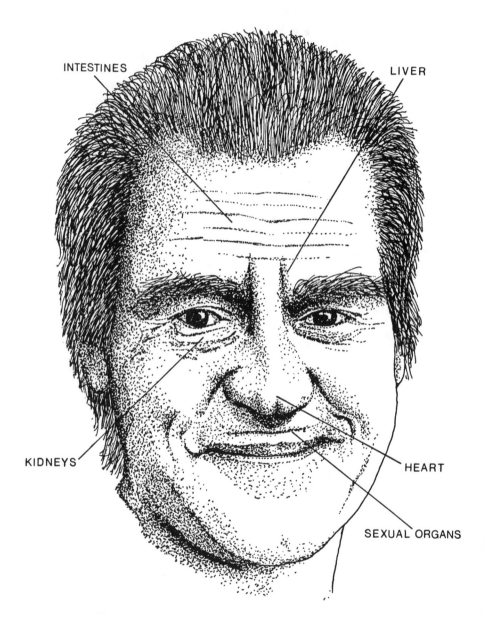

INTESTINES

LIVER

KIDNEYS

HEART

SEXUAL ORGANS

Here we can see the meaning of the most common lines that develop on the face. The depth of the lines is an indication of the seriousness of the problem.

The Eyes

To understand the relationship of the eyes to the body as a whole we must look at the evolution of Man. In the fish stage, the eyes, digestive and nervous systems were arranged in a fairly straight line. There is therefore a connection between our eyes and our digestive and nervous systems. As far as the digestive system is concerned, the eyes principally represent the liver. Many liver problems can be seen first in the eyes. As far as the nervous system is concerned, the eyes are where the system comes to the surface. They reflect the condition of the whole nervous system, and ultimately, since this system is connected to all the organs of the body, the condition of every organ.

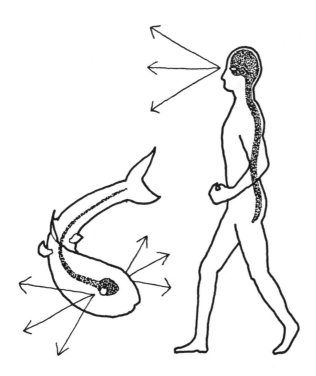

The large brain, small brain and mid-brain are placed at the top of the central nervous system, which runs down the spine, like a flower and its stem. The visual centre corresponds to the back brain in a back/front relationship. There is a similar relationship between the back brain and the liver.

The face was made by yang force, pushing from behind and causing the two sides of the face to move forward and join. At one early stage of the development of the embryo the eyes are at the sides of the head, like a fish's. If yang force was lacking during this period of pregnancy, the baby's eyes will be widely separated, showing a more yin character, lack of vitality, and a tendency towards isolation and separation in life. In the Orient such a face is called a 'widow's face'.

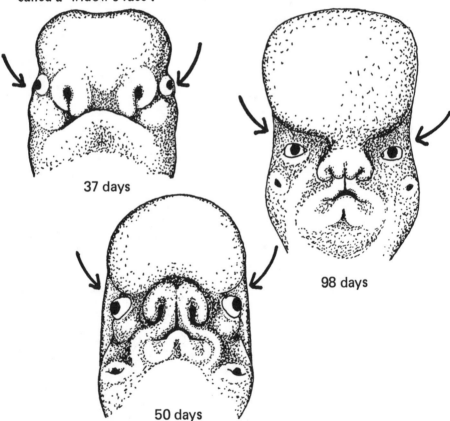

37 days

98 days

50 days

Three stages in the development of the face in the embryo, showing the contracting force that forms the features.

Sanpaku

The Japanese word 'sanpaku' means literally three (san) whites (paku). It refers to a condition in which the eye presents three white sides or areas around the iris. The usual kind of sanpaku — lower sanpaku, in which white is showing at the sides and below the iris — is caused by expansion (yin). As the eyeball becomes enlarged from excess yin, it rolls upward, since it is resting on bone and must rotate on its axis. Upper sanpaku, in which white is showing at the sides and above the iris, is caused by contraction (yang). This is why all newborn babies (who are yang) have upper sanpaku. The condition is also often found in people who are violent.

When we are becoming sanpaku in the usual sense — lower sanpaku — the whole body is becoming too yin. Instead of maintaining its desirable tautness it becomes loose — the muscles, the heart, the brain, all the organs. Practically everyone in modern society is sanpaku. Some people appear not to be sanpaku when they are looking straight ahead, but the test is whether you can see white below the iris when they are looking upwards 45 degrees. Only one in thousands or tens of thousands completely lacks sanpaku.

Sanpaku appears in proportion to the degree of the excess causing it. The more white that is visible, the worse the condition of the person.

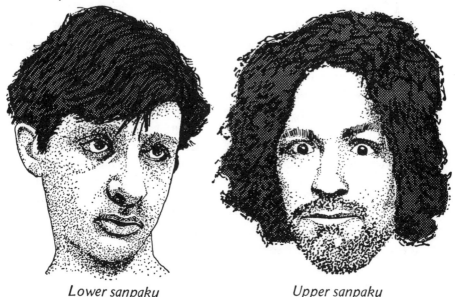

Lower sanpaku   *Upper sanpaku*

Another type of sanpaku is one in which the eyes protrude. Such horizontal expansion is less yin than the vertical expansion just discussed, but it is still a sign of sickness. When horizontal expansion occurs, the eyesight changes. The distance between the lens and the retina is altered, producing near-sightedness. The usual type of sanpaku often results in far-sightedness.

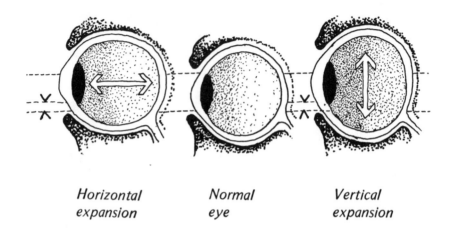

Horizontal	Normal	Vertical
expansion	*eye*	*expansion*

In the Orient both vertical and horizontal expansion are recognised as sign of misfortune or danger. In cases of sanpaku the normally compact central nerve and mid-brain become swollen, and therefore perception is not accurate. As the cells of the large brain expand, their reception of electromagnetic energies is poor. If these cells become swollen and watery, then thinking becomes one-sided, narrow or confused; the view of the whole is lost.

A healthy person has a tremendous ability to judge, and can usually sense the onset of danger. We should have this ability at least as much as animals do. Before fires in homes or wrecks of ships, rats will often escape. Snakes will dig unusually deep holes for hibernation before an extremely cold winter. Our ancestors knew how the natural environment was changing. They could tell if there was going to be a hurricane. Without listening to any weather forecast they would know several days ahead of time so they could protect themselves. These people knew the Order of the Universe and could use it. In ancient times there were many such people, but now there are few.

Your grandparents' generation included many people who knew when they would die. My own grandparents, who died in their eighties, knew several days ahead of time. They cleaned their rooms, put their private things in order, wrote their wills, visited their ancestors' graves, and prayed. None of the rest of the family knew. Then one morning they found the old people had died a natural death in the night.

Today almost no one knows when they are to die. There are assassinations — John F. Kennedy, Robert Kennedy, Martin Luther King, and countless others. John F. Kennedy did not sense his coming assassination in Texas, although he received many warnings. Because modern men and women are so often sanpaku, they are frequently subject to tragic death. People should be careful and moderate in their life, humble and modest, as our ancestors were.

Cross Eyes

Cross eyes are caused by excess yang food. In such cases the eye rotates on a vertical axis as a result of muscles contracting behind the eyes. If the eyes go in the opposite direction, towards the outside, the cause is excess of yin food. It is easy to change either of these conditions with diet. If you change to a balanced diet the eyes will move into alignment after a short time.

Round Eyes and Thin Eyes

Considering that women are apparently more yin than men, why do they tend to have rounder eyes — a more yang condition, mechanically speaking — than men? Although women tend to have a yin exterior, they have a yang interior. Here and there we get a glimpse of the yang within them. The eyes are a good example. If a woman has round eyes she will be more soft and feminine. If she has thin eyes she will tend to be more active, and perhaps masculine. A man with round eyes will tend to be more sensitive, artistic and gentle. For a man, thin eyes are a sign of a strong, active constitution.

The Eyeball

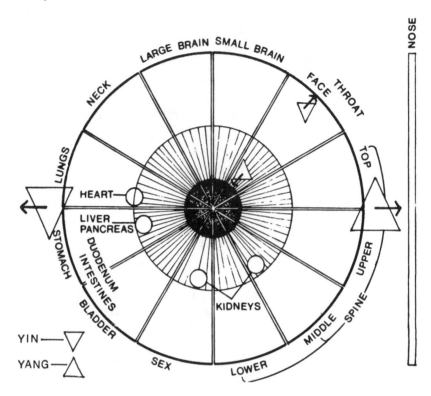

We can divide the eyeball into yin and yang areas. The yang areas are those closer to the nose and those in towards the centre of the eyeball (iris). The most yang areas correspond to the most yang parts of the body (the back). The yin areas of the eyeball are those towards the outside of the face and the periphery of the eyeball. The most yin areas correspond to the soft parts of the body (the front).

In each area of the eye the organs themselves are arranged according to yin and yang. For example, the brain is arranged from the cortex to the medula. The small brain is represented on the side of the eye nearest the nose. This part of the brain is the gathering point for nerve messages — a yang function. The cortex is represented on the outside; its functions are more abstract (yin). The intestines are arranged in the same way — the large intestine towards the periphery and the small intestine towards the centre.

If all the organs are weak, you will see twelve main bloodshot lines in the white of the eye. If there are more than six, there is serious sickness. Usually there are about four. But any lines at all indicate an imbalance in the body's condition. These lines change every day. If you eat animal products, beer, ice cream, etc. before going to bed, when you wake up in the morning you will see many small capillaries showing in the areas of the stomach, intestines and back.

If the lines end in small spots, there is hardening and stagnation in the circulation of blood or lymph. Often from looking at the area of the white of the eyeball that corresponds to sexual function you can see that the person has kidney stones. Spots in this area can also indicate problems in the lower spine or sex organs, prostrate inflammation, or cysts on the ovaries. Such spots, or dots, are usually either dark (brown or black) in colour, or red or yellow. The brown or black colour is more yin and indicates stones or cysts. The yellow or red colour indicates stagnation of blood; it is not so serious.

You can often see colours in the pupil, which should be transparent. (It is slightly blue in babies, and becomes transparent in adults.) A yellow colour indicates mucus due to malfunction of the gall bladder. A black shade shows trouble in the kidneys. Even if these colours are in a different region of the eye from their corresponding organ they have these meanings. A purple or green shade anywhere on the eye is very dangerous. Dark brown shows that the organs are becoming harder and inflexible. The eyes should have a soft translucent quality and not be hard. Hardening of the eyeball causes decreased eyesight, ending eventually in blindness. If you examine the eyes of the blind you will notice that the white part often has changed to a dark blue or grey colour.

The Iris

The borderline areas between the pupil and iris and between the iris and white of the eye indicate the condition of the nervous system.

If the boundary between iris and white becomes dim and undifferentiated, orthosympathetic sensitivity is weakening and eyesight is declining. This is common.

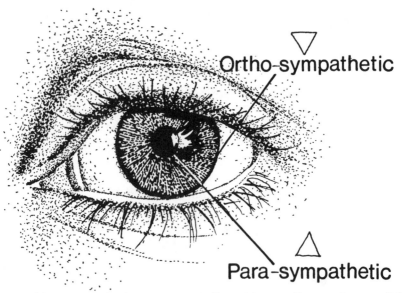

Ortho-sympathetic

Para-sympathetic

Many people have perpetually wide pupils, a yin condition, often caused by the use of L.S.D., marijuana, other drugs, or medications. The pupil should be small and respond quickly to changes in the light. If the autonomic nervous system is not working well, the response is slow and the reaction slight.

The iris is a replica of the eyeball. Dots in the iris correspond to stones or cysts or stagnated blood in the corresponding organs. We cannot see details without a magnifying glass, but we can see dots and changes in pigmentation.

Eyelids

Eyelids can be double (curving around the eyeball) or single (straight). Western peoples tend to have double eyelids, which indicates a more yin condition. Single eyelids are more yang.

The standard speed of blinking is four times per minute, or once every fifteen seconds. Blinking is a sign of excess yin. A baby does not blink at all. A healthy man's eyes can go without blinking for many minutes. If you are negotiating and your antagonist stares at you without blinking, you cannot stand it, and you lose. Cats and dogs blink more than we do. If we stare at them they look away. If you meet a tiger and stare at him, he will try to look back but finally back down. See how much a person blinks. If they blink less than you do, retreat!

The Eyelid Region

To examine the eyelids, open the person's eyes and observe the area under the lashes. This is an area of discharge. The edge, where the lashes come out, indicates the condition of the nervous system. (Hair appears at the terminal points of the nervous system, e.g. on the top of the head.) The lower lashes and lid show the condition of the sexual organs. The upper lashes and lid show the condition of the brain and head region.

Eyelashes normally slant inwards. Any curling outwards indicates problems with the sexual function. An outward slant in men indicates impotency; in women, frigidity, barrenness, or a tendency to miscarry.

By pulling down the lower eyelid and looking at the exposed area, we can see the condition of the circulatory system. This area should be pinkish. A white colour indicates anemia. (In the same way, anemia is indicated by a white colour under the fingernails when the fingers are stretched.) Sometimes the area under the eyelid is very red. This shows infection and inflammation; blood is coming to the surface. With people who eat meat, fruits and sugar, this area is often bright red. We may also see defined dots or spots in this area, which are a sign of excess yang. This condition — trachoma — is caused by animal products, especially cheese, fish and milk. Hardening is produced when the fats from the animal products are congealed by the acids from fruits or sugar.

There are tiny hollows between the upper and lower eyelids at the outside and inside corners of the eyes. White or yellow deposits here indicate mucus deposits between the organs. Deposits in the lower organs will show in the lower lids; the upper organs, in the upper lids. A yellow colour is caused by cheese and eggs, a white colour by milk and animal fats. If a woman has thick mucus there is a tendency towards vaginal discharge.

The Area Around the Eye

The area around the eye corresponds to the kidneys. Bags under the eyes are of two kinds — soft or hard — and two causes, water or fat. If a person has been drinking too much liquid, the kidneys are overworked and cannot discharge properly, so liquid accumulates under the eyes. Swelling that has a harder appearance is caused by the consumption of too many fats. The excess is stored in the kidneys as fatty deposits, which impair kidney function.

A red or purple colour under the eyes indicates blood stagnation in the kidney region, purple denoting a more advanced stage of stagnation than red. In advanced stages we can occasionally see the actual blood vessels, swollen and discoloured. In cases of swelling without discolouration, hardening is taking place; there may be stones, cysts or fatty deposits. Kidney stones are indicated by a gathering of discolouration into defined spots. All these problems appear in or around the eye on the corresponding side of the body — left eye for left kidney, right for right.

The Mouth

The mouth should be ideally about the same width as the nose — a little smaller in women. A small mouth shows yangness, vitality. A large mouth shows the opposite: contracting force was lacking in the formation of the embryo. Nowadays everyone has a large mouth. This increase in the size of the mouth is a sign of biological degeneration; it means that the digestive system is losing its strength.

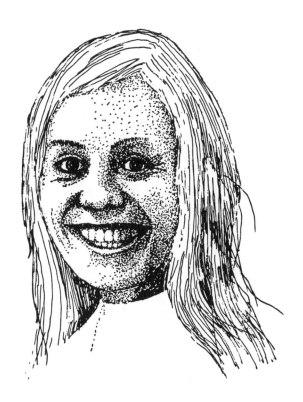

A mouth several times larger than the ideal.

The area above the upper lip (and the moustache in men) corresponds to the sexual organs. If there is a horizontal wrinkle in this area when we smile, there is weakness in the sexual organs. Such a wrinkle in men indicates weak sexual vitality, and in women, trouble with menstruation. The cause is overconsumption of animal products, including all dairy products. Vertical lines in this area show that the sexual organs are shrinking. This is commonly seen in older people who can no longer have sexual relations.

Different parts of the lips show the condition of different parts of the digestive system. The upper lip corresponds to the stomach — the top part of the lip to the upper stomach (where the strong hydrochloric acid is released), the middle part to the middle part of the stomach (weaker acid), and the lower part and the corners of the mouth to the duodenum (the exit of the stomach, connected to the liver, gall bladder and pancreas). The lower lip shows the condition of the intestines.

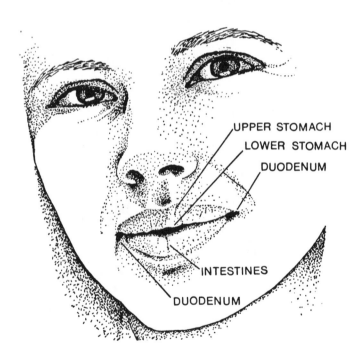

The parts of the lips and their corresponding organs in the digestive system.

If the digestive tract is expanded, flacid (yin), then the lips are swollen. An outward swelling of the lower lip shows a tendency to constipation. Dark spots or recurring sores on the lips show ulceration and stagnation of blood in the digestive system. Such spots and sores occur on the same side of the mouth as the side of the digestive system in which the irritation is present. Lips that are whitish in colour show that the blood in the intestinal region is weak, and absorption is poor. Tightness in the mouth shows that the intestines are tight (and in women, that the vagina is tight). If the intestinal villi are too tight, they cannot absorb well. But the mouth should be fairly tight, especially in women.

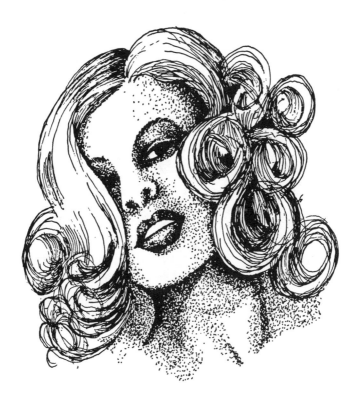

An example of example of extreme swelling of the lower lip. This is a sign of swollen intestines and a tendency toward constipation.

Teeth

In the Orient there is a proverb that separations between the teeth mean you will not see your parents when they die. A cleft in the lower lip is also such a sign. People with these features are apt to leave home at an early age and do much travelling; they will then settle down far from their parents. When their parents are old and about to die, such people are living too far away to return to them in time. The separations or clefts are caused by yin factors and can be changed by eating a more yang diet for a long time.

Teeth that protrude are yin. People with such teeth have trouble eating in a balanced way. They can understand the principles of macrobiotics, but they find the practice difficult. People whose teeth angle inwards (yang) have the opposite problem: they have difficulty in understanding the principles, but possess a great intuitive faith and find the practice easy. People who have straight teeth tend to be steady and patient. Often in modern people we see varied teeth — some teeth go in, others go out. This is caused by chaotic eating patterns, by consumption of extremes of yin and yang. People with such teeth have many problems. Their temperament, like their teeth, is varied. They become depressed or angry very easily. For them the practice of macrobiotics is difficult, especially eating in an orderly way. It takes a long time for them to find balance.

After people begin macrobiotics, the spaces in their teeth become smaller, and old fillings drop out. The fillings should not be replaced straight away. Their teeth are contracting and changing; they should wait six months and then fill them.

The Ears

The ears are located towards the centre of the embryonic spiral and so reflect the development of all three major systems of the body — the circulatory, digestive and nervous systems. The circulatory system is represented in the outer area of the ear, the nervous system in the middle ear, and the digestive system in the inner ear.

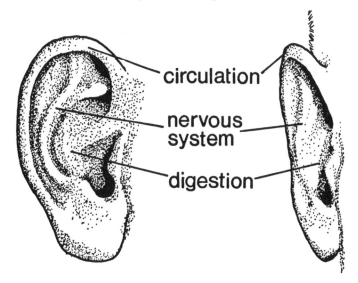

The areas of the ear and their correspondence to the systems of the body.

A protruding middle area is yang; indented, yin. The form and definition of the ear indicates what the person's mother was eating while she was pregnant.

If the ears stick out, the person has a yin constitution. A person with such ears is at a disadvantage: the radius of his hearing is not great, and he may develop a narrow viewpoint. Ears lying close to the head, especially long ones, are more balanced. The great leaders of the past all had such ears, with which to hear all sides and make sounder judgements. Small ears give a more limited perspective.

Ears that move are a sign of excess animal foods. You can see such ears on a fox or a dog.

Many older people have earlobes that are well defined and slightly detached. Detached earlobes are a sign of eating more vegetable and less animal food than most people do today. As people begin to eat more animal food, the ears become higher on the head and lose the lobes. After eating macrobiotic foods for several years, many people experience a change in the shape of the ear. The lobe will develop a fissure and detach a little, then heal up.

Hair

Hard hair means that the person has eaten a good proportion of vegetables and grains; soft hair indicates heavy consumption of animal food. Straight hair indicates consumption of more vegetables and grains, or food that is well balanced between yin and yang. Curly hair is caused by extreme yang food, or extreme yin — whether yin food or drugs. Dry hair and wet hair are caused by consumption of too little or too much liquid. Oily hair comes from eating too much animal food, especially dairy products, and from sugar.

Strong hair is the result of eating vegetables and grains in an orderly manner. Fragile hair — that is, a strand can be plucked and broken easily — is a sign of poor health.

Hair generally indicates the condition of the intestinal villi. There is actually a physical correspondence between the two, except that the villi are in liquid and the hair is in air. Baldness is a sign that our internal organs are becoming weak. We can tell which organs are concerned by the area on the head where the hair is sparse or absent.

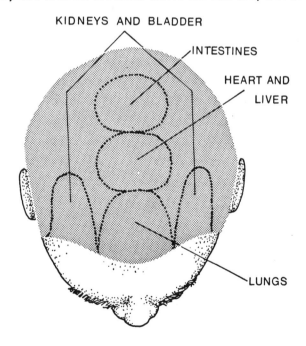

KIDNEYS AND BLADDER

INTESTINES

HEART AND LIVER

LUNGS

If for instance, someone is weakening his lungs by taking too much yin food, his hair will start to recede in the front. It is possible for the hair to grow back if the person eats wisely. Some people lose a lot of their hair when they begin eating macrobiotically, but this is only bad quality hair; good hair grows in later in plenty.

Babies, who are yang compared to adults, are usually born with light coloured hair, which becomes darker (more yang) as they grow older (and more yin). Many Japanese babies are born with brown hair, which later becomes black; then in old age, the other extreme of life, their hair becomes white (the most yin colour).

If a woman has a moustache, her reproductive organs are weakening and she probably has difficulty with menstruation. Thick moustaches on men indicate strong sex organs. If the remainder of the beard is heavy, however, it shows excessive protein intake.

There are generally two types of hair: so-called baby hair, which is silvery and fine in texture, and normal adult hair, which is darker and coarser. Baby hair on the body of an adult indicates overconsumption of milk or other dairy products. Such baby hair does not appear at random, but lies along the meridians and also the paths of connecting tissue and muscle. We can think of this as an overflow of protein from the organs. If there is trouble with the kidneys, for instance, then baby hair will appear over the kidney region; hair on the chest indicates weak lungs.

Excessive body hair is caused by eating too much protein, either directly as protein, or indirectly from excess food which is converted into protein. Even if you have cut down on your intake of protein — especially animal protein — if you are overeating you will retain excessive body hair.

The Skin

Skin Colour

Colours can be seen on the body in two ways: as specific features, such as spots, dots, lines, etc., or as a general colouration. The yang colours (brown, red, etc.) have a tendency to gather into specific features. The yin colours (yellow, green, etc.) tend to be more diffuse.

Each colour that appears on the skin indicates a certain condition of the body. The colours of our environment are the green of plants, the blue of the sky, the white of the clouds. We came from these natural colours; we make balance with them. Therefore the healthy human body does not have these colours — it has colours *complementary* to them. If we drink milk, for example, we take on the colour of clouds; we begin to have nature's colours. We are returning to nature, our origin; decomposition and death are approaching.

Red

The colour red can appear in three ways: as a general colouration, as spots, or in the form of individual expanded blood capillaries. Red skin indicates a yin condition: the heart is overworking, causing the expansion of the capillaries towards the surface of the skin. In the early stages of the problem the capillaries are still soft enough to produce only a general colouration. But eventually the arteries and blood vessels harden and the capillaries themselves appear on the surface. The cause of these conditions is excess yang — animal food, including fish, and also salt. A pink colour rather than red is produced by the addition to red of white from milk consumption.

On some occasions, however, veins come to the surface naturally. One such time is pregnancy, when a woman's body undergoes enormous activity. The peripheral parts of the body become more yin as the centre becomes more yang through activity in the depths of the womb. The surface expansion causes the veins to appear. After pregnancy a woman's skin should become very clear and clean. If she was consuming yin foods, however, this does not happen, and the surface of the skin is spotted with the dischage of these yin factors.

Blushing is normal. It indicates an active circulation. Becoming red quickly upon drinking alcohol is also a good sign. If you become warm and red after drinking only half a glass of beer, your condition is very good. A pale or grey colour after drinking indicates deep sickness.

Brown

Brown is generally a sign of trouble with the liver and gall bladder. The colour brown can appear as a general colouration (including tanning) or as spots (freckles). It can also be caused by consumption of white rice or monosodium glutamate, which is often added to foods in processing. A quite different cause of brown is excess salt. The two different processes are sometimes called 'sugar burns' and 'salt burns'.

If the mother eats very yin food during pregnancy, it will show up on the baby as a 'birthmark'. The location of the mark tells us which organ is affected and at what period of the pregnancy this excess occurred. With good eating, birthmarks can fade but seldom disappear completely.

Yellow

The colour yellow is an indication of problems with the pancreas, liver and gall bladder. We can see this phenomenon most clearly in jaundice, where the person's whole colouration becomes yellow — even the eyes. When bile cannot flow normally it moves into the blood instead of the duodenum. In the blood it is carried through the entire body. For such an over-yang condition we should eliminate the over-yang foods — salt, meat, etc. — and include more vegetables. Sometimes a person eating macrobiotically can develop this skin colour by eating too much salt.

Newborn babies are small and yang; a slight yellow colour is normal. Mother's milk makes them progressively more yin, and they lose this yellow colour. Babies sometimes have jaundice. This is not normal, but understandable if the mother has been eating excess animal food.

Green

The colour green is seldom seen, except in very yin parts of the body such as veins. Green is seen in nature as the colour of the plant world, in the form of chlorophyll. The colour of the animal world is red, in the form of haemoglobin. Man's essence is red. If green appears on the skin — except in very yin places such as the veins — it is a sign that our animal quality is degenerating and regressing into a vegetable quality. A greenish cast to the skin is typical of people suffering from cancer, the major degenerative disease in the Western world. A slight green colouration indicates a tendency to develop this disease.

If you observe the people on the streets you can see many with this slightly green shade. It occurs mostly on the sides of the face, indicating lung cancer, or on the back of the hand between the thumb and index finger, indicating cancer of the intestines. This colour also appears frequently on the stomach meridian on the legs. The expression 'green with envy' is very appropriate. Cancer patients tend to be irritable, pessimistic and sometimes greedy; people with such dispositions do in fact tend to be more susceptible to cancer.

Blue and Purple

If the veins, which normally appear greenish, become more yin through intake of refined sugar, cold drinks, soft drinks, ice cream, etc., the green colour changes to blue or purple. This is a very dangerous sign. We rarely see blue, but purple is quite common, especially among older men. Many men over forty develop red or swollen noses, and sometimes a purple colour appears. The red colour is caused by the expansion of the vessels, but purple indicates a more advanced stage of degeneration. Purplish colour on the nose indicates a very expanded heart and high blood pressure. When the heart starts to become expanded, more pressure must be used to pump blood; that is high blood pressure. When the heart expands even more, it begins to lose its force; low blood pressure is the result, and the veins appear purple. A purple colour is even more dangerous than green. In cancer death usually comes slowly. But although a person with a purple colour may appear active and healthy, death can strike at any moment.

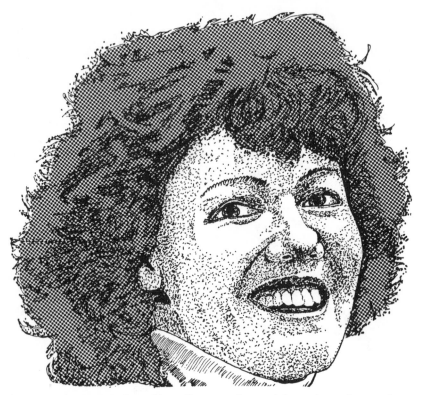

A nose which is red and swollen on the end is a sign of an enlarged heart and an overburdened circulatory system.

Black

On the body the colour black can appear as spots or dots, or as a general colouration over a wide area. This colour is often associated with kidney problems. The cause is usually extreme yin, especially strong medication and drugs, or cold yin foods or drinks. The cause is yin, the colour is yang. Black is the colour of death. In tuberculosis patients we see a very pale colour; as they approach death their skin colour tends toward black.

Sometimes we find black spots, or so-called beauty marks. These occur mostly on the acupuncture meridians or on the junctions of muscles or connective tissues. By noticing which meridian they lie on we can deduce which organ is in trouble. They often appear after a high fever, when the sickness has run its course.

When we were born we had no beauty marks and very clear skin. Therefore beauty marks are a record of sickness and fever while we were growing up. If we eat wisely for a considerable time, these marks can fade, but they never disappear completely. Moles, which are more brown in colour and caused by excess eating or an excess of animal protein, can disappear completely, especially if we avoid overeating.

Grey

A greyish cast to the skin is quite common in Western industrialised countries, though it is seldom found among people who eat wisely. It indicates a swollen, hard liver. The skin is insensitive and dull. People who have this grey colour are often easily depressed ('grey') and tend to become angry. Although this colour is similar to black, it does not occur in spots, but appears as an overall colouration.

Pallor

Pallor indicates a yin condition in the lungs. Again, there are no spots or dots: it is a general colouration. There may be asthma or other respiratory problems, including allergies.

Transparency

A transparent and pale quality of the skin can be seen in people suffering from tuberculosis or skin diseases caused by bacteria, especially leprosy.

White

A white tinge to the skin, especially a milky shade, is very common nowadays, because of heavy consumption of dairy food. It appears both as spots and as a general colouration. Sometimes the white spots appear much the same as freckles, particularly on the lower leg, forearm and upper back. In such cases, the cause of the spots is still dairy products, but more yoghurt and cheese (especially cottage cheese). In a healthy person the complexion has a slightly white colour, but the quality is different than the dull white caused by consumption of dairy food. In health the skin is firm and tight and radiant. The Japanese word for a healthy complexion is OMOSHIROI, which also means 'interesting'. The characters that make up the word are those for face or surface (OMO) and white (SHIROI). Traditionally the Japanese people realised that if individuals' faces were white, they were leading healthy, happy, interesting lives.

A General Comment
Different racial groups have different underlying skin colours, but the same characteristic colours appear in all people suffering from disease; we just need to train ourselves to see them. With black people, for instance, we can see the colours most clearly in the hands, faces and eyes.

Skin Texture
Each individual's skin also has a unique texture: smooth, rough, oily, dry, etc. Each texture indicates a certain condition.

Rough
The skin of most people in the West is generally smooth until they are about twenty to twenty five years old. After that age the skin rapidly becomes rougher (yin). This condition is caused by excess animal fats. An abundance of saturated fats in the diet produces a hard texture in the skin.

Oily
Oily skin results not only from eating too much oil, but also from overeating. When we overeat, the excess food is converted into fats, which come out on the skin as oil.

Wet
Excess liquid on the skin indicates overconsumption of water or other drinks. We can feel this condition when we shake hands. People like this sweat easily, and their feet and underarms are often damp. They are suffering from overburdened kidneys and sometimes an overworked heart.

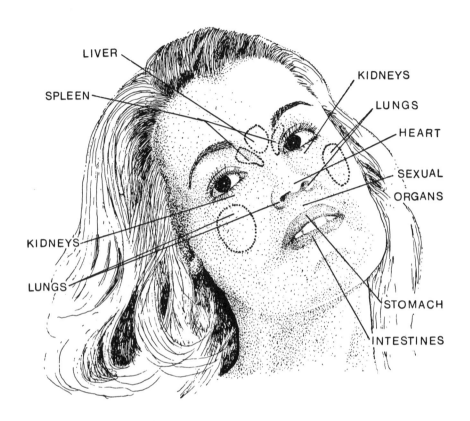

LIVER

SPLEEN

KIDNEYS

LUNGS

HEART

SEXUAL

ORGANS

KIDNEYS

LUNGS

STOMACH

INTESTINES

The above areas of the face are used for spotting problem in the organs concerned. Abnormal colours, changes in the texture of the skin, or surface eruptions or rashes are early signs of developing problems.

The Hands

The wrist of a healthy person is flexible enough to bend backwards at a 135 degree angle without any pain. If it will only go forwards 90 degrees, hardening is present.

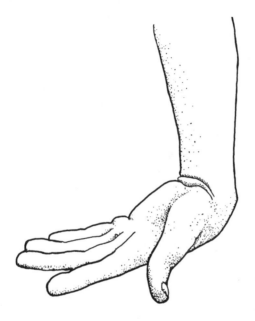

The wrist should be able to bend backwards 135 degrees without pain.

Make a fist and push between the knuckles. If you cannot make an indentation between the knuckles, there is hardening of the arteries and the kidneys are swollen.

Hold the fingers out straight and see whether they are straight or curved. Straight is normal. If they are curved check to see which meridian ends or begins on that finger (see chart of meridians on p. 53). Curving away from the thumb is yin, and towards the thumb is yang.

Next, look at the length of the fingers. The middle finger is the longest. The index finger and ring finger are often different in length. If the index finger, which represents the intestines, is longer than the ring finger, it indicates that the intestines are quite yin. A longer ring finger shows that the triple warmer (metabolism) is yin. Left and right hands are not always the same, indicating problems in the left and right sides of the body.

Hold your fingers straight and together; see if there are any holes betweeen them. If there is space between the fingers, you are yin, and therefore somewhat impractical; money 'passes through your fingers'. The fingers should be tight together (but not swollen). Swollen fingers are an indication of high blood pressure.

The tips of the fingers show the top of the body — the brain. The lower parts of the fingers show the sexual organs. If the fingers are red, purple, painful, and if the nails are chipped, broken, or weak, the ability to think and the generation of sexual energy are poor. An enlarged top section of the finger, like a snake's head, indicates a very yang constitution. The person was originally yang at birth but consumed excess yin, which led to expansion of the periphery — fingers, toes and nose. Often people with such fingertips have difficutly getting along with others. Their inner character is tender, but their rough manner of expression repels people.

Check the joints of the hand for hardness, swelling or arthritis. In cases of real arthritis the joints will become painful, and each section of the hand will become swollen or tight. Women have a greater tendency towards swelling of the hands. If a man's hands start to swell he is usually eating or drinking too much. His kidneys and heart are becoming swollen and weak.

Lines on the Hand

With the thumbs together and the palms out, you can see the totality of the hands. The lines in the hands form a spiral.

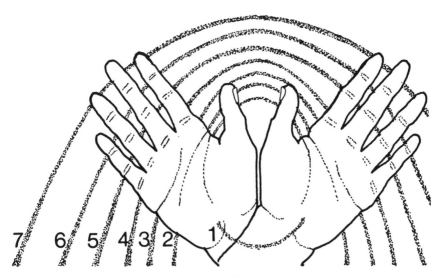

The spiral structure of the lines of the hands.

For our purposes we need only pay attention to the four principal lines in the hand, which in the West are usually called the Heart, Head, Life and Fate lines.

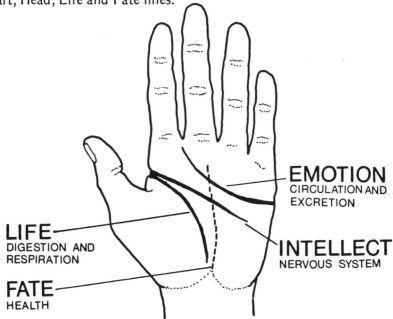

EMOTION
CIRCULATION AND
EXCRETION

LIFE
DIGESTION AND
RESPIRATION

INTELLECT
NERVOUS SYSTEM

FATE
HEALTH

The four principal lines of the hand and their physiological correspondence.

These lines should be seen as representative of their corresponding organs. The so-called Life Line represents the digestive and respiratory systems. This line, the first circle of the spiral of the hands, is around the base of the thumb and encloses the area corresponding to the intestines — the fleshy mound below the thumb. Stiffness and pain in this part are a sign of intestinal problems. The length of the Life Line can be broken into a logarithmic progression corresponding to the years of one's life, as shown in the diagram below.

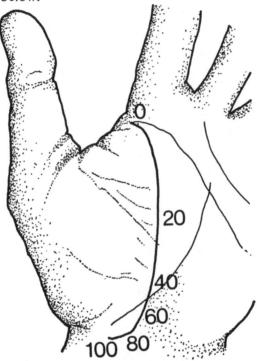

The positions of the Life Line corresponding to the age of the person concerned.

To the middle, it shows up to the age of about twenty. The part to the junction or fork (if there is one) shows up to forty-three to forty-five. And so on. Ideally, this line should be very clear and long, going all the way round the bottom of the hand. If it is doubled, the mind is also split; around the corresponding age there will be social and mental difficulty. If the line is jagged and unclear, the digestive and respiratory systems are weak, and sickness may occur at any time. A break in the line indicates that there will be danger, serious sickness or death. Through proper eating one can change these lines; a broken line can join.

The Line of Intellect corresponds to the nervous system. This line should also be strong and clear. If the nervous system is more yin and the person tends to be intellectual, the line tends to go downwards and be longer. With a more yang nervous system the line tends to be shorter and go straight across or slightly upwards. People with such lines are active and practical, rather than artistic and romantic.

The Line of Emotion corresponds to the circulatory and excretory systems, which include the heart, kidneys and bladder. A long line extending towards the index finger is a sign of yin. It is better if this line goes to the mount below the index finger. Some people have another line, the Line of Love, a horizontal line which shows above or across the Line of Emotion. It indicates an emotional or poetic nature.

The Fate or Destiny Line is another line which only some people have. It is a vertical line going up the centre of the palm. It shows that your mother was hardworking and that you have a strong constitution.

Nails

If the nails (usually on the index and middle fingers) turn white when you stretch your fingers, you are suffering from anemia. White spots indicate consumption of excess sugars or fruit. Since the nails grow continuously, they are a record of what we have eaten. The portion closest to the cuticle shows your eating pattern a few weeks ago; the middle portion corresponds to three to four months ago; and the top, about six months ago. Of course, the rate of growth varies somewhat with each person. As we grow older our nails will take about nine months to grow from base to top.

In young people the half moon which shows at the cuticle is a good sign. It is yin, and young people need yin to grow. After the body is mature, the half moons gradually lessen, until after the age of thirty-five they should slowly disappear, leaving only a small trace.

Long nails indicate a yin constitution; short, square nails, a yang constitution. In heavy drug users the nails become rough, with broken tips. This indicates sexual problems and confused thought processes. (The region between the thumb and index finger of people who take many drugs also becomes purple, indicating intestinal stagnation).

General Comment
Wide hands with short fingers indicate a relatively yang, more active constitution. Narrow hands with long fingers indicate a relatively yin, intellectual or artistic person. The strength of the hand grip shows the person's vitality.

Touching

The Meridians and The Pulses

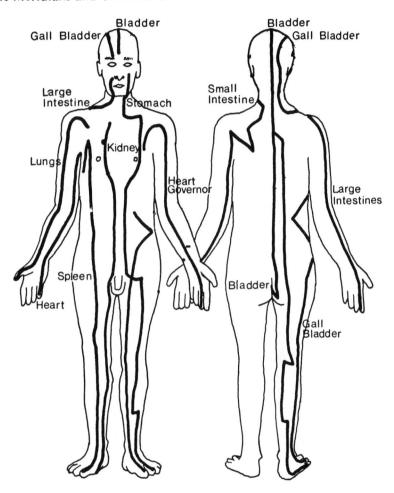

The Meridians

Ki or Ch'i energy — also called prana, orgone energy, etc. — circulates through the human body in fourteen channels or meridians. Ten of these meridians correspond to organs or specific functions of the body: bladder, gall bladder, heart, kidneys, lungs, large intestines,

liver, stomach, small intestine and spleen/pancreas. Four of them correspond to more general functions: governor vessel, conception vessel, heart governor and triple warmer. (For more details on the meridians see the books on acupuncture listed in the bibliography.) The principal meridians are shown in the drawing above.
below.

A knowledge of the meridians is useful in diagnosis. For instance, moles, spots, warts and discolouration occur along the meridians, indicating problems in the corresponding organs. A good test to discover which organs are weak is to apply pressure to main points on the meridians. If an individual feels sharp pain when you press a point, the corresponding organ is weak. A few such points are shown in the drawings below.

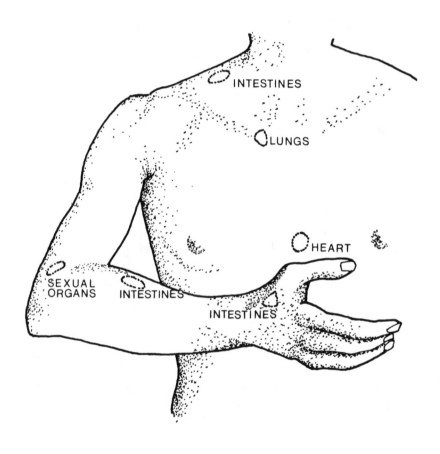

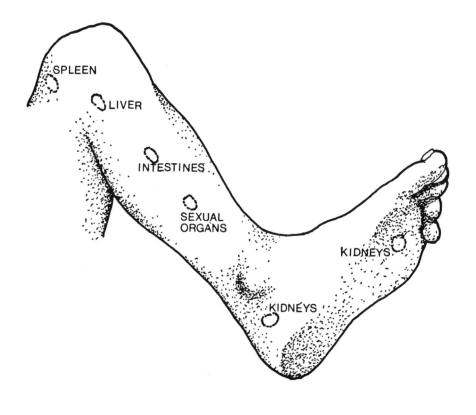

SPLEEN

LIVER

INTESTINES

SEXUAL
ORGANS

KIDNEYS

KIDNEYS

In addition to points on the meridians we can look for areas where there is swelling or stiffness, discolouration or excessive body hair. Some of these areas are on the meridians; some lie over the organs themselves. The following two drawings show several such areas on the front and back of the body.

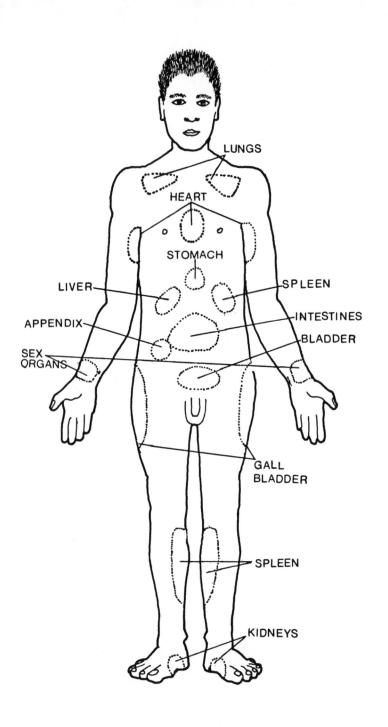

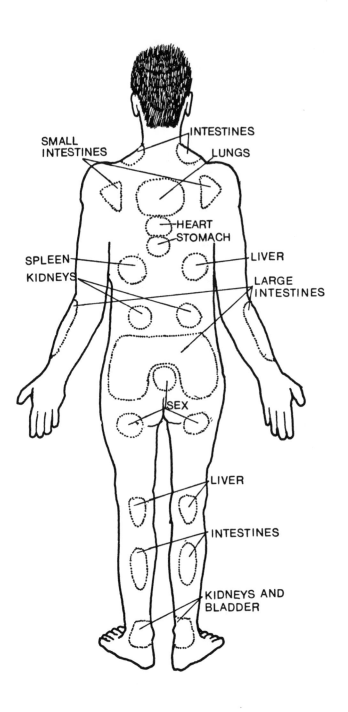

SMALL
INTESTINES

INTESTINES

LUNGS

HEART

STOMACH

SPLEEN

KIDNEYS

LIVER

LARGE
INTESTINES

SEX

LIVER

INTESTINES

KIDNEYS AND
BLADDER

The Pulses
Western medicine recognises only one pulse. Oriental medicine recognises three on each wrist, each of which can be taken on the surface or by pressing deeply. The pulses and their corresponding organs are as follows:

Right Hand
1. Deep: Lungs
   Surface: Large Intestine
2. Deep: Spleen/Pancreas
   Surface: Stomach
3. Deep: Heart Governor
   Surface: Triple Warmer

Left Hand
1. Deep: Heart
   Surface: Small Intestine
2. Deep: Liver
   Surface: Gall Bladder
3. Deep: Kidneys
   Surface: Bladder

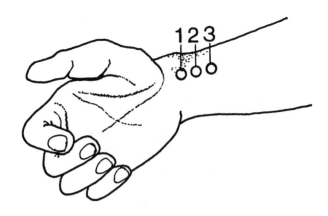

The surface pulse is felt by light touching; the deep pulse, by deeper pressure, firm and constant, although not so much as to cause pain. After some practice you can learn to find these pulses easily. The exact line of the pulses depends on the person concerned; you have to search to find it.

The surface pulses correspond to the yin organs (bladder, gall bladder, large intestine, small intestine, stomach, triple warmer), and the deep pulses to the yang organs (heart governor, heart, kidneys, liver, lungs, spleen/pancreas).

When taking pulses hold the person's hand lightly with one hand. Use the index, middle and ring fingers of your free hand to feel the pulses. Start from the bottom fold of the wrist; then each finger will fit into the proper place. It is best to close your eyes and keep very quiet. Practise by taking the pulses on yourself. You may find that one or two of the deep pulses are missing. If four or five are missing, the person's condition is critical.

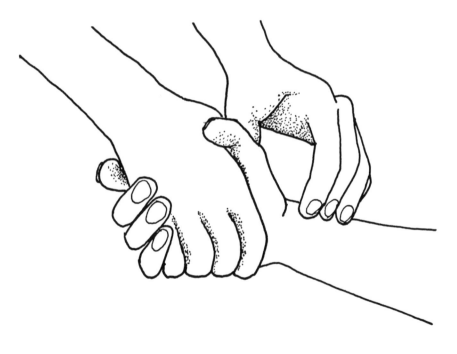

The position of the hands taking the pulse.

I myself rarely take pulses. When I do, I feel *in between* two of them. This shows the correlation between the antagonistic/complementary organs represented by each pulse. For instance, the pulse between the kidney (deep) and bladder (shallow) positions shows the condition of the kidney/bladder system. This is not a traditional technique, but I find it very useful.

The pulse on the front of the throat indicates the state of the whole mind and body. A slow, steady, quiet pulse indicates calm spirituality; a pulse that is racing or uneven shows mental disturbance.

The Voice

Hearing

Judging a person's condition by hearing requires a more refined sensitivity than judging by sight or touch.

Everyone uses one ear more than the other to listen with. The favoured ear is the one closer to the centre of the spiral pattern of hair growth on the head. Hearing is most acute through the sector parallel to the axis of the spiral. People tilt their heads to one side or the other depending on where their spirals are located. A spiral on the right side of the head indicates that the person's mother had a stronger constitution than his or her father, and vice versa.

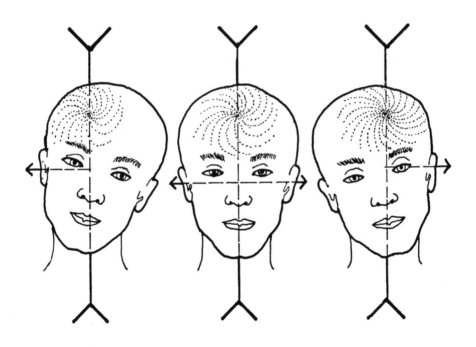

Voice Qualities

We can gain an idea of the condition of people's internal organs by listening to their speaking voices. The pitch of the voice is regulated by the lungs, its speed and rhythm by the heart. Other qualities can be recognised by very careful listening, and by comparing different people's voices. When listening, use the antagonisms: high/low, fast/slow, loud/soft, sharp/dull, dry/wet, clear/unclear, penetrating/not penetrating, tense/loose, regular/irregular (stuttering). Some of these antagonisms are discussed below. Try to work out the significance of the others for yourself.

High/Low. A high voice is produced by very contracted vocal cords. When a man becomes an adult his Adam's apple expands; his voice therefore changes from high to low. Because a woman's Adam's apple is more contracted, her voice is higher. Salty foods and refined carbohydrates make the pitch of a voice higher. Water, dairy products, oil and fat make it lower.

Fast/Slow. A fast voice is more yang. A yin person speaks slowly, especially a sick person. Most mentally ill people speak slowly, although certain yang mental illnesses — hysteria, for example — are characterised by fast speech.

Loud/Soft. If a voice is not firmly rooted (coming from deep within the body), the intestines are functioning poorly. Some people have very weak voices; it is difficult for them to speak or read aloud. As well as showing shallow breathing — and therefore bad lungs and infirm intestines — this characteristic often indicates a very yin autonomic nervous system.

Dry/Wet. A wet-sounding voice is a sign of excess liquid in the body, moisture in the lungs, and overworked kidneys. Sweating, swollen legs, diminishing sexual activity, an enlarged heart, thin blood, expanded capillaries, and falling hair are all conditions that can accompany a wet voice.

Clear/Unclear. An unclear voice is caused by mucus in the throat.

Handwriting

In order to judge people's conditions by their handwriting, examine personal letters rather than business letters. The first thing to notice is the general character of the writing. Is it pleasing to look at and clear to read? Next, observe the details: the slant of the letters, whether forward, backward or straight; the regularity of the spacing between the letters; the consistency of the height of the letters; whether the written lines have a tendency to slant upwards or downwards on the paper.

Here are two examples of handwriting. Which is yin and which is yang?

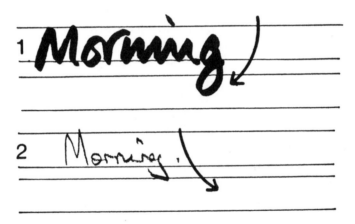

The forward slant of the first example is more yin; the backward slant of the second example, more yang. Handwriting with a vertical direction is more balanced. It is difficult for children to write with a forward slant — they are too yang. Women, however, tend to write with a forward slant.

Lines that slant upward are yin; lines that slant downward are yang. Vertical strokes are yin; horizontal strokes are yang. In English, yin strokes predominate; yang strokes are used mainly for connecting. In between are the circular strokes, which can be either yin or yang, depending on their form.

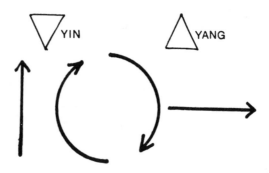

Yin people coordinate the rhythms of their writing with their breathing. Yang people coordinate it more with their heart beat. (In general, speaking is in harmony with breathing, and writing with the heart beat; but there is a tendency for yin people to be influenced by the rhythm of their breathing when they write.)

The spoken word is more yin than the written word. A yang person is drawn to speaking; a yin person, to writing. It is difficult for a yin person to speak in front of many people: he will prefer writing. Very few people can do both; most people have a preference. Among great religious figures in history, for instance, Jesus was very yang, so he wrote nothing, but Confucius was yin, so he did a great deal of writing.

When we begin to write, consciousness (yin) comes first, and also the will (yang) to write; these are complementary, front and back. Then intellect begins to work — seeing that there is no misspelling, seeking clarity, etc. — and also determination. Then comes emotion — the desire to write beautifully, to be artistic — and sentimentality. Then follows sensory desire, and modification. Finally, we want to reach the end, to complete the task, which is an expression of our more mechanical nature.

All of these aspects of our judgement succeed one another at enormous speed. These five stages occur in each word, each sentence, paragraph and chapter. The influence of the organs of the body on these aspects of judgement is as follows:

——————————————————— BODY ———————————————————

Head	Lungs	Heart	Intestines	Nerves
Brain	Breathing	Circulation	Sexual function	Reflexes
1	2	3	4	5
Consciousness	Intellect	Art	Sensory desire	Instinct
Will	Determination	Sentiment	Adjustment	Completion

——————————————————— MIND ———————————————————

Even one word, one sentence shows this order. A handwritten communication that is regular at the beginning and irregular towards the end indicates that the writer's intestines and autonomic nervous system are in poor condition, although the brain, heart and lungs are functioning efficiently. With this tool we can see the overall condition of the people who write to us, and whether they are practical, romantic, cold or warm — as well as many other things about their character and state of health.

Habits

All individuals have a unique, characteristic way of presenting themselves which is an indication of their internal condition. For instance, they may make certain habitual gestures while talking. These signs are messages that can be used to diagnose the mental, physical and spiritual condition.

Many habits are acts of self protection by the body. The outer structure of the body contracts, expands, bends, or twists to accommodate and make balance with internal disturbances. For example, if the lungs are functioning poorly, the shoulders will move forward to protect them. Sometimes people cross their arms — just as in their mother's womb — to make themselves more yang. They do so because the inside is yin and weak. If mucus is scattered throughout our lungs, we feel more safe and secure with our arms folded across the chest. Crossing the legs is also a telltale sign; it shifts the weight off one or the other side of the intestines.

We are all different; we each have our weaknesses and strengths. One person may be attracted to art; another may not. We may be attracted to playing music, but if our fingers are stiff we will content ourselves with listening. A person with small eyes tends to enjoy a relatively yang form of art such as home decorating, which requires more physical activity than writing, for example.

A person who was born yang and attracted to yin foods is more apt to develop into a spiritual teacher, artist, etc. Those who are born yin and attracted to yang foods tend to become more active as politicians, businessmen, lawyers, etc. Our selection of work can tell much about our constitution and condition. The same is true of our selection of friends, lovers, husbands or wives. One man would never even think of marrying a certain woman; another man may fall in love with her immediately. We are all seeking balance through polarity.

Advice on Food

Proportions of Foods

In the Beginning, the earth was composed of elements and simple compounds — hydrogen, oxygen, nitrogen, carbon dioxide, water — and from these life began. Protein molecules were formed, building primitive cells. Then two main lines of development evolved, one yin and one yang: the plant kingdom and the animal kingdom. In the diagram below we can see how these two channels developed simultaneously and complementarily.

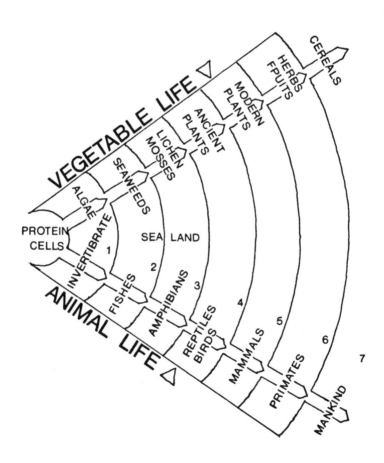

Humanity is the terminal point of this 3.2 billion year evolutionary process. As a species, humanity evolved and has continued to survive by eating cereal grains, which appeared on the earth under the same climatic conditions as we did.

The evolutionary process develops logarithmically with time. To determine when each period of development took place, we can divide the total 3.2 billion year period by two, then divide that sum by two, and so on.

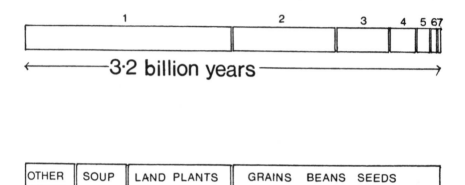

The first scale shows the periods of evolution. The second scale shows the proportions of food in a proper diet — which are complementary to the time proportions. In other words, half of the diet would be made up of cereal grains, beans and seeds, the most recent foods to evolve. Half of the remaining portion would be land vegetables. Then half of the remaining portion would be sea vegetables — including soup, which is a replica of the ancient sea we evolved from.

The unit of division in this logarithmic progression can be changed, but the principle remains the same. The proportion of main food should be decided first; then the secondary foods will follow the logarithmic progression. Here are two examples.

50%		25%	12%	
GRAINS		VEG.	SOUP	OTHER

70%		20%	6%
GRAINS		VEG.	SOUP

Food proportions, showing how the change in principal food changes the total diet.

If you begin with 50% of the total for the staple food, then 50% of the remainder is the next category of food, and so on. If you begin with 70% for the main food, then the next category is 70% of the remainder (70% x 30% = 21%), and so on. People who are suffering from a condition due to excess yin need to become more yang. To accomplish this we expand the proportion of main food (cereals), which will make the other proportions smaller in relation to the total intake of food. If the person is too yang, then the reverse is true: decrease the proportion of cereals, which makes the proportions of the other foods correspondingly larger. When you advise someone on diet, start with the appropriate percentage of cereal grains, and work from there.

The Order of Eating
Thorough and proper chewing is extremely important. It aids the digestion of all foods, but especially of grains, which are digested almost entirely in the mouth rather than in the stomach. Remember the saying: Chew your liquids and drink your solids. And merely moving your jaws up and down is not enough. Use your molars efficiently: chew in a circular or spiral motion.

It is not advisable to eat near bed time. If you do not leave three or four hours between eating and retiring, food will sit in the stomach and intestines while you sleep and will not be digested properly.

A meal is best eaten from yang to yin. Grains are the main food, so we take them throughout the meal. We go from soup to vegetables, and if there is fruit we end with that. The main food is balanced, but the side dishes have mixtures of yin and yang. There may be many different vegetables, but even if they are cooked together we should eat the yang ones (root vegetables, etc.) first, then proceed to the more yin ones (leafy greens, etc.) always alternating with grains. (See the food table on p. xiv.) Since salad is yin it should be eaten toward the end rather than the beginning of a meal. A salty soup comes at the beginning of the meal (the salt stimulates digestion), but a 'sweet' soup should be taken at the end. Yang beans such as aduki beans can be eaten throughout the meal along with the grains; yin beans such as soya or lima beans, at the end. If you eat yin foods before the meal, your appetite is decreased and your meal will not 'sit' well. Even if you are eating good food, it will not be effective unless you consider the order of eating.

Salt

Since salt is yang, with a more yang diet the amount of salt is increased; with a more yin diet the salt is decreased.

Many people trying to eat macrobiotically are unnecessarily afraid of salt. They do not wish to become yang. Life is a process of expansion, growing towards death and extreme yinization. This same life process also creates sickness and decomposition. If we expand, yinize, too quickly, we destroy ourselves. Modern humanity seeks extreme yin in the form of sugar, coca cola, ice cream, etc., and is destroyed. To be more yang — to decompose more slowly — and to govern our lives in moderation is the secret of longevity. Do not seek to be lazy and comfortable. Even though taking salt is difficult, use it to keep the process of life slow.

Because many young people today have taken a lot of drugs, making their autonomic nervous systems weak, they have lost their innate judgement and cannot control themselves well. Such people need smaller amounts of salt, to be increased gradually. Several years ago, people who were starting to eat macrobiotically could use quite a bit of salt and not have any bad reactions.

Now people who enter macrobiotics are weaker and need to be more careful; they cannot change so quickly. It is amazing to see such a big difference in just the last six or seven years. After a period of yangization through good eating, we are free to begin experimenting with food to become more yin or more yang, as we choose.

Animal Foods

If we wish to eat animal food it is wiser to choose those animals that lie furthest away from us on the evolutionary scale. Of all the animal foods, fish is the most commonly used in macrobiotic cooking. Although the animal kingdom is generally more yang than the vegetable kingdom, fish is not necessarily yang. Depending on the type and method of cooking, it can be yin or have yin elements. The small dried fish that still have the bones (Japanese iriko) are yang. However, the white fish often served in restaurants can be quite yin. Fish is a good source of protein. Protein is yin. Therefore salt or tamari (soy sauce) is used in cooking fish. Instead of thinking, "I ate fish and became yang", it would be more correct to think, "I ate fish *with salt* and became yang". The point is that animal foods contain certain qualities of both yin and yang; we must use them carefully.

Giving Advice

Giving advice entails not only telling a person about treatment for their particular condition, but the physiological, mental or psychological, and spiritual causes of the condition. If you begin and end with symptoms you are a 'professional', a specialist. You should try to help people remember their infinite dream, together with the understanding that this world is ephemeral. Symptoms can be cured and eliminated, but ultimately people have to understand their total freedom and their own creation of their misery. Without such understanding they will repeat their sickness and come back to you. When you treat sick people try to set them on the path of rediscovering their innate freedom. It is difficult, but possible. You can, of course, use specific treatments and local applications, you can eliminate symptoms, but that should not be your purpose. Do not limit yourself.

The greatest difficulty with giving advice is that even though you may understand the cause of a person's problems, you have to communicate that to them effectively. If the person does not practise what you suggest, then your effort is in vain. But if you can see people's wholeness — the unity of physical, mental and spiritual condition — you can communicate with them in a way they can understand.

If a person is egocentric, only seeking self gain, you may have to say that they had better see a specialist, that this is not the place for them. Many people seek only personal, selfish gain. This mentality has made them sick. If you cannot turn their mentality around 180 degrees, their health and happiness will never be secured.

To erase symptoms is easy, but to change a person is difficult. You can see a few hundred patients and become a good symptomatic doctor. But to turn people toward freedom you must see thousands, and this is a lifetime's training — perhaps the training of many lifetimes, I do not know. Our diagnostic advice is primarily *education*. Its purpose is to develop the sick person's view of life, his spiritual, mental and physical condition. This way of healing was practised by Jesus and Moses, but there are very few practitioners of this holistic medicine among the millions of doctors in the world today.

There is no word to describe a practitioner of this kind of medicine. When I first met George Ohsawa, I wanted to introduce him to some professors at Tokyo University, where I was a post-graduate student. I needed some personal history and asked him what I should write about his occupation. He could not say. He was not a doctor, or a nutritionist, but more — something like a philosopher, yet not in the academic sense. George laughed at my perplexity, and I always laugh when I have to write my occupation. For it is a way of life, not categorised. Many students want to learn Oriental medicine. They say "I am an acupuncture doctor", or "I am macrobiotic", but that is ridiculous, if you think about it; a person is not limited, confined, to anything. If we know the Order of the Universe, we are limitless.

When you give advice you will find that there are two kinds of people: (1) those who see only the small view, the details, and neglect the whole; (2) those who see the big view, but are not keen on detail. We must give opposite kinds of advice to these two types of people. With the first type, you tell them, for example, how to cure a tumour with application of compresses, etc., then you go to the cause — why the tumour arose. You lead their thinking to their way of eating, then to their way of thinking. "You trust modern medicine too much". Or, "You are too egocentric: that is why you ate the foods that led to this sickness". For the second type of person this approach must be turned around. They may say, "Probably I made a mistake — it is my karma", not talking about their tumour or other symptoms. You must therefore lead their thoughts from the whole to the parts. "Yes, your sickness came from karma. But what is karma?" You should explain that karma is the Order of the Universe. Then explain what they should eat within that Order, then finally discuss their symptoms.

You must learn to understand the person's level of judgement. There will be some people who come to you with fragmentary knowledge, talking about, say, vitamin B12 and other modern concepts. When they ask advice, begin at that level. Unless you start at their own level, they will not be able to understand. You must explain to them in scientific terms the effects of the food they eat, and how they need to change it.

You have to train yourself to be very flexible. Staying at one level is not being a free man; if we stay at a very high level all the time, that is being a saint. A limitless person goes freely from one level of thinking to another, according to the circumstances. To do this we must loosen our rigidity, become friends with everyone, and have the same loving feelings for everyone. Then we can give advice to all kinds of people. If there is someone or something you dislike, you are still limited, and your ability to give advice is decreased. If Richard Nixon should come to you for advice, say, "Hello, Richard, what is the trouble?" Do the same with a sick animal: "Hello, rabbit, what is the problem?" For anyone, the same. A free person acts like that.

You cannot stay with a sick person all the time. You must respect a person's freedom to the maximum; if people really want to die, let them: it is their freedom. The point is never to become an authority figure; remain a friend or adviser. People should not come back repeatedly for consultation; if they do, your advice has been incomplete — you did not know how to give them proper advice about freedom, the cause of causes. If they do not understand that, sick people become slaves; they are still afraid inside, and are dependent. That is no way to build a healthy world and help people become happy and free.

Two types of people are easy to help: (1) People who have experienced the range of fear completely and now want to be free. They have tried many different symptomatic approaches and been disappointed. They are now ready to give up their defensive way of life, their stubbornness and their rigidity to find freedom and regain their health. (2) People who have specific ailments but still retain a strong spirit. These people had a strong biological base embryologically and in early childhood, even though they spoiled their health in later life. They have a base of commonsense and appreciation — which they have forgotten. They only need to be reminded.

Individuals' ability to cure themselves depends on whether they have a strong will. This internal faculty can be seen by the following diagnostic signs: (1) a large head; (2) firm bone structure, especially with men; (3) eyes that remain focused firmly when the person is talking. People with these characteristics can do what they are determined to do.

The essence of macrobiotics is our ability to live in harmony with the order of nature. To see whether people can follow a macrobiotic way of life, look for signs of order in their constitution and present habits. The first sign of a potentially well-balanced sense of judgement is teeth that are straight and well formed. Next observe the vertical balance of the body. Imagine a vertical line running down the middle of the body and see if the two sides are generally balanced. Then do the same with the front and back of the body. See if the arms hang vertically at the sides, if the nose is straight or slants to one side, and if the ears are vertically aligned to the head. See if the spine curves. A large curvature generally makes it more difficult for a person to develop balanced judgement.

Next check the horizontal lines. Balanced eyebrows are a good sign, as are balanced ears and straight shoulders. It is natural for these lines to be a little off balance, but the more they are off the more difficult it will be for a person to maintain balanced judgement. Next look at the curved lines: the collarbones, rib cage, pelvis. When standing, the angles of the feet should be roughly equal. It is best if the feet are straight ahead, but if the feet angle to the inside or outside, they should do so equally.

Consider the orderliness of individuals' personal manner and lifestyle. Do they arrive on time? Do they slam the door? If people live with respect for others, keep their things in order, wait to eat with others at the table — these are indications that they are thinking of the whole and not just of themselves. If we see ourselves as simply part of the larger whole, then we can create happiness in our lives and those around us. An orderly person can understand macrobiotics very easily; more narrow people need time and patience until they can understand basic causes.

Orderliness appears psychologically as an attitude of appreciation or gratitude. Much of this mentality is nurtured in childhood. If a mother is sloppy, her children will have a tendency to be sloppy too. From our mothers we learn the differences between social and selfish behaviour. The most difficult people to change are those who were given too much rich food in the womb and in childhood and received excess knowledge, techniques and concepts from modern education. With such people you must be very patient. The first step is to change their diet, which will help to change their mentality; then start to discuss with them ways to recover their own freedom. Sometimes you must give a hint and let them do the rest by themselves. Often George Ohsawa would say to a patient, "Figure it out for yourself". These people were always making appointments and hanging around him, causing him many troubles, but he wanted them to be truly free whether he lived or died.

If people do not understand what Infinity is, our advice becomes symptomatic or conceptual. We have seven principles and twelve theorems (see p. ix   ). Please study them until you master them. The key is to let people understand this Order of the Universe. That is our foundation.

For more information on East West activities; East West centers in your area; or other books in the Macrobiotic Home Library series, call or write to:

Kushi Foundation
P.O. Box 1100
17 Station St.
Brookline, MA 02147
(617) 731-0564

Suggested Readings

Aihara, Cornellia. *Macrobiotic Kitchen: Key to Good Health.* Tokyo: Japan Publications, Inc. *The Do of Cooking,* 4 vols., Oroville, Calif.: George Ohsawa Macrobiotic Foundation.

Dufty, William. *Sugar Blues.* New York: Warner Publications.

East West Foundation. *The Macrobiotic Approach to Cancer,* Wayne, N.J.: Avery Publishing Group, Inc.

East West Journal. Monthly. Brookline, Mass.: East West Journal.

Esko, Wendy. *Introducing Macrobiotic Cooking.* Tokyo: Japan Publications, Inc.

Esko, Edward and Wendy. *Macrobiotic Cooking for Everyone.* Ibid.

Kohler, Jean and Mary Alice. *Healing Miracles From Macrobiotics.* Englewood Cliffs, N.J.: Parker Publishing Co.

Kushi, Aveline. *How to Cook with Miso.* Tokyo: Japan Publications, Inc.

Kushi, Michio. *The Book of Do-In.* Ibid.

Kushi, Michio. *The Book of Macrobiotics.* Ibid.

Kushi Micho. *Macrobiotic Dietary Recommendations.* Brookline, Mass.: East West Foundation.

Kushi, Michio. *Macrobiotics: Experience the Miracle of Life.* Ibid.

Kushi, Michio. *Natural Healing through Macrobiotics.* Tokyo: Japan Publications, Inc.

Kushi, Michio. *Visions of a New World: The Era of Humanity.* Brookline, Mass: East West Journal.

Ohsawa, George. *The Book of Judgement.* Oroville, Calif.: George Ohsawa Macrobiotic Foundation.

Ohsawa, George. *Cancer and the Philosophy of the Far East.* Binghamton, N.Y.: Swan House.

Ohsawa, George. *Guidebook for Living.* Oroville, Calif.: George Ohsawa Macrobiotic Foundation.

Ohsawa, George, *Zen Macrobiotics.* Ibid.

Ohsawa, Lima. *The Art of Just Cooking.* Brookline, Mass.: Autumn Press.

The Writers

About The Author

Michio Kushi was born in Kokawa, Wakayama Prefecture, Japan in 1926. His early years were devoted to the study of international law at the University of Tokyo, and an active interest in world peace through world federal government in the period following the Second Wold War. In the course of pursuing these interests, he encountered Yukikazu Sakurazawa (known in the West as George Ohsawa), who had revised and reintroduced the principles of Oriental medicine and philosophy under the name "macrobiotics." Inspired by Mr. Ohsawa's teaching, Mr. Kushi began his lifelong study of the application of traditional understanding to solving the problems of the modern world.

Mr. Kushi came to the United States more than thirty years ago to pursue graduate studies at Columbia University. Since that time he has lectured on Oriental medicine, philosophy, culture and macrobiotics throughout North and South America, Europe and the Far East; he has also given numerous seminars on macrobiotics and Oriental medicine for medical professionals and personal counseling for individuals and families, including many cancer patients. While establishing himself as the world's foremost authority on the macrobiotic approach, he has guided thousands of people to restore their physical, psychological and spiritual health and well-being as a fundamental means of achieving world peace. He has also presented an address to a special White House meeting and two addresses to the delegates of the United Nations on the applications of macrobiotic principles to world problems.

Mr. Kushi is founder and president of the East West Foundation, a federally-approved, non-profit, cultural and educational organization, established in Boston in 1972 to help develop and spread all aspects of the macrobiotic way of life through seminars, publications, research, and other means. He is also the founder of Erewhon, Inc. the leading distributor of natural and macrobiotic foods in North America, and of the monthly *East West Journal* and the quarterly *Order of the Universe* periodicals. In 1978 Mr. and Mrs. Kushi founded the Michio Kushi Institute of Boston, an educational institution for the training of macrobiotic teachers and practitioners, with affiliates in London and Amsterdam; and at the same time, as a further means toward addressing world problems, established the annual Macrobiotic Congresses of North America and Western Europe. A non-profit organization, the Kushi Foundation, was established in 1981 to assist with the coordination of educational and research activities.

Mr. Kushi's published works presently include *Natural Healing through Macrobiotics, The Book of Macrobiotics, The Book of Do-In, How to See Your Health, Oriental Diagnosis, Visions of a New World; The Era of Humanity,* and the quarterly *Order of the Universe.* Mr. Kushi presently resides in Brookline, Mass., with his wife Aveline and children.

About The Editors

William Tara has been presenting the macrobiotic approach to health via public lectures, seminars for medical professionals, and personal counseling throughout Western Europe and the United States for over fifteen years. He is the founder of the Michio Kushi Institute and the Community Health Foundation in London, and is currently serving as the Executive Director of the Kushi Institute in Boston.

David Lasocki studied chemistry at University College in London before coming to the United States, where he studied music history at the University of Iowa. He has been studying macrobiotics since 1971.

About The Illustrator

David Elliot studied architecture at Manchester University and the Architecture Association in London. He has studied macrobiotics since 1970, works as a freelance design consultant and architect, and teaches Hatha yoga.

Index